Bombs, Boils & Brushes ...

... a Rural Doctor's Notes

Dr R. J. Robertson

The Shetland Times Ltd.
Lerwick
2008

Bombs, Boils & Brushes ... a Rural Doctor's Notes

ISBN 978 1 904746 37 9

First published by The Shetland Times Ltd., 2008.

Printed and published by
The Shetland Times Ltd.,
Gremista, Lerwick,
Shetland ZE1 0PX.

Contents

Acknowledgements

This rather simple story is the result of telling the more amusing stories about life as a country G.P. in Shetland to many friends, who frequently suggested I write a book. I eventually took their advice and jotted down some of those yarns.

This would never have been completed in a form people could read if it had not been for my daughter, Jane Manson, who coped with the illegible writing and produced a typed copy for the publisher.

I would like to dedicate this book to my long suffering wife Maureen and to the many fine patients in both practices who made life so pleasant for me.

2008

Life's but a walking shadow, a poor player,
That struts and frets his hour upon the stage,
And then is heard no more.

Macbeth – William Shakespeare

Chapter 1

The first eleven

I HAVE some pre-school recollections but they tend to be like vague flashes from a dream, totally unconnected but I presume based on reality: a heap of sand with a tip-up lorry, a black cat, some vague faces without names and a pop-gun brought back from Aberdeen as a present. A pop-gun, for younger readers, had a cork on a string; it fired the cork a few feet by air pressure.

The earliest things I can remember with some clarity relate to primary school days at the Infant School in Lerwick, that is the old Infant School at the south end of King Harald Street. Time plays tricks on our memories and it appeared to me then that we, the infant pupils, had to stand in twos at the back of the hall of the school for an infinite length of time in absolute silence. In reality, it only happened once a year on Remembrance Day and only lasted two minutes. Of course, it was a penance without comprehension at the time.

I remember the teachers mainly as faces. There were two Misses Angus and they are very vague as I was not taught by either of them and they appeared quite old to me. Mrs Deyell and Miss Blance both did their best for me though I did not do my best for them. I know there was some parental involvement, possibly due to an inability to sit still and therefore a lack of attention.

I have no recollection of moving up to the Central School, it was all just school I suppose, but I would have been there when the first bit of excitement occurred as I would have been seven. At that time we lived at the Meteorological Observatory out the South Road, above the Waterworks at Sound. I came to school with some sort of transport in the morning, probably by car with my father. Later on there was a school bus which came from as far away as Quarff. In the summer at a later stage I walked home but to start with went to my grandfather's house in King Harald Street after school and was picked up from there at tea time.

On the day of all the excitement I was walking along King Harald Street with all the others when planes appeared from the north, flying at roof-top height parallel to the street. We were fascinated and I remember waving to what I took to be the pilots, clearly visible in the transparent noses of the planes. I protested when this interesting display was rudely interrupted by a relative who yanked me out of the street into the house. It was only much later that I understood the reason for this curtailment of my pleasure. These were Heinkel 110s which had bombed a seaplane in the North Harbour and set it on fire. The 'pilot' was the nose gunner and it was fortunate that they did not fire on the people in the street, most of them being children.

My grandmother who lived in King Harald Street was a rather stiff, imperious, unapproachable woman and was very conscious of her social status in the town. Afternoon tea parties were common, attended by ladies of a similar social strata so I caused some consternation on arriving from school there one afternoon. One lady remarked on my 'sleek', and how smart it was. I innocently replied it was not a 'sleek', but something on my hair for nits.

When I got a bit older, I walked back from school with my great pal Alex Younger. Alex lived just below the Waterworks in one of the very few houses at Sound in those days. He was much better versed in the ways of the country than I was and the journey home in the afternoons took a long time. Time was meaningless to us once we were free from school, there were so many diversions on the way home and we rarely walked along the road.

I was introduced to a game called 'Kick the Block' at Sound. I don't know if this game is still played by children in Shetland or if it was purely a game played in that area, but it was really a type of 'Hide and Seek'. The seeker had to guard the block, which could be an old tin can or similar turned upside down, and the hiders tried to creep back towards the block unobserved in order to kick the block before the guard could touch you. It was played in an area with plenty of nearby cover. If you were seen at a distance the seeker ran back to the block and kicked it and put you out; only when within a regulation circle round the block did you have to be touched.

We all had 'hurlies' and the Sound brae was ideal for these. A rudimentary brake was essential on that hill although the ditch usually ended the run. The brake consisted of a stick which was pivoted and could be pulled back against one of the wheels. Pram wheels were much sought after and the competition fierce. Alex had linoleum on his hurlie I remember, the old fashioned brown stuff. It could not have helped him to stay on board, especially if it got damp. It all goes to show how little traffic was on the South Road in those days.

Occasionally, Dr McKenzie had to come to the Observatory to see a patient and he had a grey/silver Brough Superior. We boys were quite fascinated with this car, the only one of its kind I have ever seen.

There did not seem to be any football in those days and Alex and I backed different bus companies. As far as I can remember there were only two. Alex backed Ganson's and I was a supporter of Tait's. We argued the pros and cons of the two companies for ever.

There was an initiation test at Sound known as the 'Big Leap'. Until you had done this you were not really one of the gang. It consisted of jumping from a high rock on one side of the Sound burn, across a deep pool to a grassy bank at a much lower level. It appeared dangerous and risky to me but, of course, Alex could do it with ease and I had to follow suit or lose face, so I plucked up the necessary courage and did it only to discover it was relatively easy. I have never explored the Sound burn since and don't know if it still exists as a burn or what has happened to it in the mass of houses now built in that area.

I don't know how our gas masks stood up to the rough and tumble on the way back from school. They were issued in a brown cardboard box about six by four by four inches. Everybody acquired a cloth bag with a strap which fitted the box closely. I don't think I had to carry a schoolbag in those days but the gas mask had to be carried always.

About this time, when I lived at the top of the hill, we boys were treated to aerobatic displays over Lerwick by Gloster Gladiator biplanes from Sumburgh. We were thrilled to watch them loop-the-loop etc., and were very proud of them. Little did we know that these obsolete aircraft formed the fighter defence of Shetland and were completely outmatched by the modern aircraft of the Luftwaffe. Undoubtedly, these aerobatic displays over Lerwick were visual propaganda exercises, which seemed to have the desired effect.

From then onwards my school days revolved around the war, of which there was shortly to be much evidence in Lerwick and throughout Shetland. As we grew older, maps were essential so that we could follow the war elsewhere and we listened to the news and noted advances, retreats, victories and defeats, and knew all the personalities involved. Most of us schoolboys could indicate the position of the various armies on a map, believing every word from the BBC and being too immature to see through what was not broadcast. Of course, there were no daily papers at that time that I knew of.

Military camps sprang up all over the place and the 'Circus Park', in the centre of Lerwick where the Up-Helly-A' galley is burned now, became an army camp, right opposite my grandparents' house. Bren gun carriers appeared in Shetland, another fascination with their erratic, jerky steering. I doubt if they would have been much use if there had been an invasion but they impressed us schoolboys and as there were never any tanks it was the next best thing.

Tank traps were built out the South Road and out the North Road. These consisted of large square concrete blocks or concrete pyramids, about a foot and a half high. A new road was constructed parallel to the North Road called Cunningham Way and is where the present North Road now runs. What had originally been the road north went off to the right at the end of the Ladies' Drive, ran down into Dale and climbed steeply to join again at the Windy Grind. This track was improved and a wooden bridge put across the Dale burn. I presume these roads offered alternative routes in case of bombing but I never really understood their rationale.

I now lived in Lerwick and was much nearer the centre of activity. There was a derelict house somewhere about where the top of Gilbertson Road now is and it was surrounded by barbed wire. At that period there was little in the way of housing in that part of the town so this two-storey house stood all alone. I was very impressed by this place as it was the 'glass house' for military defaulters and we boys observed it from a safe distance.

The main centre of interest was the harbour front and as it was open young eyes saw most of what went on. It was imperative that the harbour had a twice daily visit, if possible, or at least after school in the afternoon. Troopships, large heavy lift cargo vessels, submarines, corvettes, frigates, destroyers, boom defence vessels, steam drifters, launches, air sea rescue launches, Norwegian refugee boats and, later, submarine chasers for the Norwegians, were just some of the ships and boats to be seen round about the old Fish Market, built of red brick and faced with white tiles and now replaced by Alexandra Building. The Fish Market was all naval offices. There was a torpedo store and workshop at the north end of the market where LHD had their wire store. This establishment always had its doors wide open and schoolboys were never chased off by the sailors who worked there.

The submarines normally berthed at the north end of the market, nearest to the torpedo store. They were mostly British with one or two Norwegians, a French one called *Minerva* and one Polish one. I remember these, but there may have been others. The Jolly Roger flying from the conning tower of a submarine coming into the pier was noted, and any white bars on the flag which denoted kills. Now and again a submarine would be open to the public and, of course, no prizes for guessing who was front in the queue.

We knew all the flags of the allies and also their national anthems which were played on Saturday night on the radio.

Boys always collect something and instead of cigarette cards or stamps or whatever is in vogue, at the time we collected military badges. There were numerous regiments based in Shetland and we collected them all: Black Watch, Camerons, Highland Light Infantry, Green Howards, Seaforths, Royal Engineers, Pioneers, King's Own Scottish Borderers, to name some of them. There was somewhere in Lerwick where these could be purchased and I think it was Laurenson Bros. on Commercial Street. Any other war material was collected and great pride taken in bits of shrapnel, cartridge cases and other junk. I had an Orlikon cannon case at one time and it was unique.

The Anderson Educational Institute was taken over as a military hospital and I believe the boys' hostel became naval headquarters. This meant a reshuffle of Institute pupils into the Central School which then over-spilled into various rooms in the town, so my classroom was in the Methodist Church basement for a period. I remember it because there was a shop which sold sweets, where George Robertson the electrical shop is now. Anything we could buy was either a cheap substitute or on ration.

Another time the class was in an upstairs room in the now redundant United Free Church at the top of Church Lane. To end my Central school days I went to the Bruce Hostel. The 'prep' or homework room downstairs on the left was used as a classroom. When I had to go there it fitted in perfectly with the harbour front both morning and afternoon. By this time I was living in Commercial Road.

A little later in the war Mitchell's Yard, in the road past the Malakoff, was used as a storage area for bits of aircraft waiting for shipment south. Sometimes a complete fuselage of a Spitfire would be found there and our imaginations ran riot sitting in the cockpit of the wreck. The machine gun button was on the joystick and could be pressed in imaginary air battles, always accompanied by a loud impersonation of a machine gun. It had to be taken in turns to 'fly' this fighter having executed a commando penetration raid to reach the wreckage. There were no notices that this area was out of bounds, but there was suspicion in our minds that is was. This added to the excitement of the adventure.

Perspex rings became all the rage about this time. If the raw material was available, and there was a constant supply of broken bits at Mitchell's Yard, then they were easy to make but difficult to polish. A knife and a file were the tools and something like Vim cleaner for polishing. Looking back, I cannot understand what the attraction was because boys did not wear rings and girls were something we put up with, so I don't think they were ever the recipients of these crude ornaments.

I was particularly lucky as my father's firm did all sorts of repair on ships and often damaged warships limped into Lerwick to be patched up sufficiently to make the rest of the journey to dry dock down south. This gave me the chance to go on board some of these ships with him. I can remember being on board HMS *Eclipse*, a destroyer which had received a torpedo in the engine room and had been towed into port. Looking into the engine room I saw it was a mass of tangled wreckage and full of water. A patch was made for the hole and the compartment pumped out before she was towed away.

There was a sloop, HMS *Pelican*, which lay at the south end of the fish market and had either torpedo or mine damage aft. The entire after section of the ship stood vertically in a twisted mass though the remainder of the hull appeared intact. There was a lot of activity round this ship with divers cutting and clearing up some of the mess. The senior diver working on the *Pelican* was a naval man, a chief petty officer called Davidson. He was well known to us and many others in Lerwick at that time, being a ruddy faced, broad shouldered, real tough nut. The story was told at that time that Davidson stayed down for much longer than the usual diver and particularly so after lunch. He did not seem to move so much as others either. These divers wore the old diving suit with the diving helmet and piped air from a hand pump on the pier. A rush of air bubbles from the release valve on top of the helmet rose steadily to the surface and so the position of the diver under the water and his movements could be guessed at. Apparently, having had a liquid lunch, this experienced diver could wedge himself up against a face underwater, regulate his air supply to give him negative buoyancy then have a sleep. Meanwhile, the pump men turned the handles on the air supply. These pumps had a man at each handle and it was quite hard work to pump for any length of time so normally they were spelled.

There was a strange destroyer with four funnels in the harbour called the *Saint Mary*. I was on board it at one stage as it had also received some damage. She was one of fifty American destroyers of an earlier vintage given to Britain by the USA at the height of the Battle of the Atlantic when things were going so badly for us.

Another attraction of going aboard these naval ships was milk chocolate. I was always given a bar or two of this chocolate and it was very precious at that time because sweets were not only rationed but much reduced in variety.

Two things which I missed during the war from the food point of view were bananas and Puffed Wheat. When Puffed Wheat made a reappearance after the war I thought I had dreamt the stuff existed and was delighted to find it was real. I still like it better than any of the breakfast cereals.

Not only did we boys know all the cap badges of the various regiments in Shetland, but we knew all the badges of rank in their proper order. This was actually of some benefit to me later when I did my national service as the different salutes required for different ranks in all three services never posed any problem for me, though remained a mystery to many of my colleagues.

Living in Commercial Road did have one alarming but exciting episode. The Norwegian navy had a base where the HIB factory was built at the foot of Brown's Road, directly below our house. I was in bed with infective hepatitis at the time and remember clearly some bustle and excitement in the house as a Norwegian motor torpedo boat had gone on fire and ammunition was exploding. I was rushed out of bed and taken up to King Harald Street. There was considerable anxiety as the boats carried depth charges or torpedoes and there was some fear of them exploding also. All the residents in the area were evacuated. The story goes that the boat was shelled by another naval vessel to make it sink and one Norwegian sailor, who was sleeping it off below, was quite unaware of the fire until a shell made a large hole in the space where he slept. Reputedly, he calmly dived out of the hole and swam ashore.

I did not actually see Norwegian refugees coming ashore but did see the boats which they had escaped across the North Sea in. Again these fishing boats or small steamers were of great interest to us. One sank at the north end of the market after arrival at Lerwick. She was later salvaged and became, I think, the *Roerwater*.

My father had a steam drifter during the war, and a motor boat. The drifter was the *Maid of Thule* which had a very nice sheer to her hull and was one of the more handsome drifters around. She was transformed by a large gallows which projected out over the bow and a heavy mast set immediately in front of the wheelhouse with a heavy derrick. I can remember going to the old whaling station at Olna with my father to look at a heavy winch, probably used for hauling whales up during the life of the whaling station. This winch was refurbished and set in front of the mast. These necessary alterations did not help the beauty of her lines but made the job of lifting seaplane moorings much

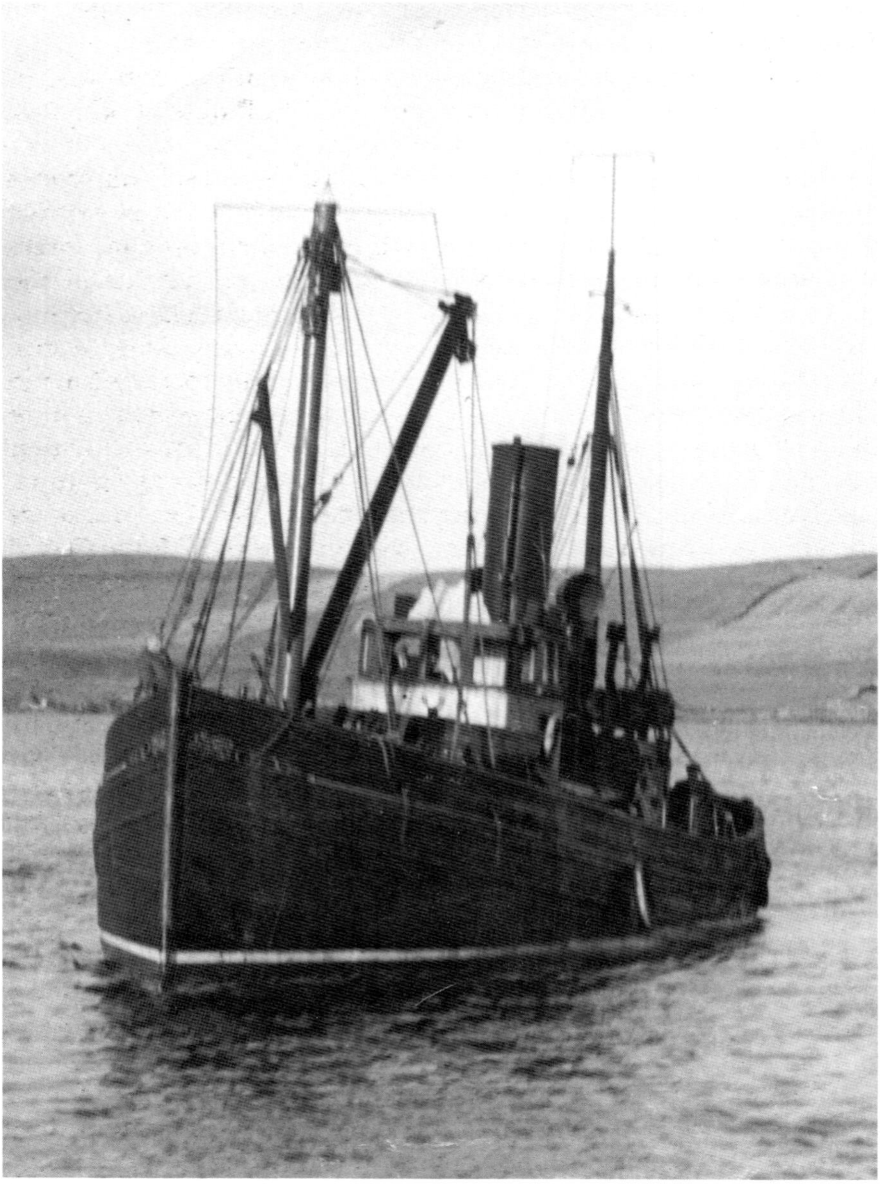

S.D. Gossawater *in heavy lifting guise.*

easier. The motor boat was the *Trust*, later to become the *Laxowater*. The *Maid of Thule* became, after the war, the *Clingswater*. There is an interesting photograph of both vessels lying in the small boat harbour in A.T. Cluness' book *The Shetland Isles*.

I spent a lot of time round and about these vessels on school holidays or on Saturdays. On Saturday mornings I acted as office boy in my father's office. I earned a shilling for running messages and doing simple tasks. The three people I remember in the office were very good to me: Margaret McLeod who later became Mrs Jack Keddie; Jessie Martin (nee Murray); and Andy Beattie whom I used to meet occasionally and swap old stories with. On one occasion I had to 'run a message' to Holmsgarth, where Burgess' garage is now. It was a fairly long walk for me at that time and my destination was a large hut used pre-war as a gutters' rest hut and, probably, first aid station, run by the Church of Scotland. At this stage of the war it was some sort of Home Guard headquarters and my message was for Sir Arthur Nicolson of Brough Lodge in Fetlar. He was a Home Guard colonel or similar if I remember correctly. Anyway, he spoke very nicely to me and gave me half-a-crown. To anyone who does not know what that is, it was two shillings and six pence; I earned one shilling for my Saturday job so I felt very well rewarded for my long walk.

The Home Guard used the building immediately above the new premises built by Home Furnishing and still occupied by them. I think the original business was in the Home Guard building. Andy Wilson, who was the gas works manager and lived in that aromatic residence known as Gas Cottage behind the gas works, was the sergeant-major in the Home Guard. He was remembered by me because he had access in the NAAFI to fruit squares, an unknown treat in those times. He would bring some of these along to our house from time to time.

Some younger readers will not remember the gas works. It was a smelly establishment built on the bend of Commercial Road where Charlotte House is now. The effluent from the gas works came out at the gas pier, now disappeared under the new fish market. The gas pier was a convenient, if somewhat malodorous, place for boys to sail home-made boats. These consisted of a piece of wood for a hull, a bit of galvanised metal stuck into it as a centre board and keel, and a mast with a paper square sail. Not only did the gas works outflow discharge here, but also that of the slaughterhouse in Harbour Street. Sometimes it was the 'Red Sea' down there, but it never seemed to cause any health problems to us.

Fishing for sillocks along the various piers and on board fishing boats lying there was another popular way to spend our holidays, albeit not so popular with mothers when we came home. The equipment was simple – a bit of brown 'skoag' and a few hooks from Jamie Irvine's shop (where D. & G. Leslie's is now), then 'rick' a sillock or two for bait to catch the rest. Unless there was a cat at home the results were thrown back into the harbour.

Holidays at that time were spent at home but we did have a couple of weeks in the country once or twice, on two occasions at Snarraness, West Burrafirth and at Irvine's Hotel at Spiggie. At that age I enjoyed the Spiggie ones much better than the Snarraness holidays. There was always some other young company at Spiggie, but none at Snarraness.

Most of the Sinclair family were at home at Snarraness and, during the summer, Dr Jamieson and two medical students. The students laboured with stones and cement to make jetties and landing places in front of the house during the day and spent the evenings studying anatomy with Dr Jamieson. The latter wore a skull cap which intrigued me and I was told he made the students drink out of moustache cups. Having learned how to skull a punt in the small boat harbour in Lerwick, I learned to row a boat at Snarraness, but apart from that I felt it was a bleak, unexciting place, relieved by the odd evening at the fishing, especially setting a long line and the expectation of what the next hook would bring up on hailing it. We always went back to fried flukes for supper.

One day my father was going to row a boat to Sandness and take me with him. He asked Dr Jamieson how long it would take, and got the answer: "It all depends how much you intend to carry." It was many years later as an anatomical student myself that I came across Jamieson's plates. These were coloured plates of anatomical dissection used by most medical students and compiled by the same Dr Jamieson. I was told he could have been Professor of Anatomy at Edinburgh University but would never accept the post.

Saturday afternoons were always spent at the pictures. The North Star ran a matinee performance and I went whatever the film being shown. Often it was a western, which suited us fine. The top idol of the day was George Formby with his ukulele, followed close behind by Laurel and Hardy, Abbott and Costello and, on a few occasions, the Marx Brothers. All the war films were closely followed and games modelled on them.

Sundays tended to be rather depressing, mostly because there was Sunday school. I hated it for more than one reason, but mainly because it was boring. I can never be certain if the Sunday school teachers did it because they believed they had a mission to perform or whether it was their only chance to control others and mount a platform. Certainly they required a lot of lessons themselves if they wanted to transfer any of their messages across to children. Not only did my two sisters and myself have to attend each Sunday, but had to get dressed up to do it. There was also the loss of freedom, albeit only for an hour or so. In descending order of penance it was boredom, followed by having to get dressed up, then the confinement.

At least once or twice during the war I flew to Aberdeen with my parents. Shetland was a restricted area and you had to have a permit to leave it or to get back in. The terminal at Sumburgh consisted of two small huts set on the grass just beyond the end of the Tolob road. One belonged to Allied Airways and the other to Scottish Airways, the two companies operating at that time, who flew De Haviland Rapides. These were small, two-engined biplanes which carried about seven people. It was always cold, in fact very cold, on these flights - no pressurised cabins in those days - with little gaps in the door where the cold air screamed in. There was a strict weight distribution among the passengers; we were all weighed before take-off and being a youngster I was allocated the rearmost seat as less weight allowed the tail to rise easier on take off. The windows were blacked out on these small planes and I can remember sitting with one eye screwed to a scratch in the blackout all the way to Aberdeen. What a reliable and, in retrospect, safe service these small planes gave before and during the war.

I was fascinated to see the first aircraft after the war at Sumburgh because they were German troop carriers requisitioned at the end of the European war; Junkers three-engined aircraft with one engine on each wing and the third mounted on the nose of the plane. They were made out of corrugated metal to add to their unique appearance. I never flew in one but saw them start up on a number of occasions and the flames always shot out from behind each engine as it started. Eventually, after a fairly short time, they were replaced with Dakotas.

I was up at Sullom Voe once or twice during the war with my father who had responsibility for the aircraft moorings in the voe. I can still recognise the position of the guard room on the approach from Brae well out the Scatsta road. A pass was required to get past this outpost but surely schoolboys were considered harmless as I got in. Sunderland and Catalina flying boats were the aircraft involved. On one occasion one of these aircraft jettisoned her depth charges at her mooring. As these were activated by a pressure pistol dependant on depth they were relatively dangerous and had to be recovered. 'Johnnie the Diver' did the diving for this job and received official recognition from the Air Ministry for his part in it. Johnnie was a first cousin to my grandfather and along with Robbie Robertson, a brother to my grandfather they were the two divers in Shetland in those days, although Robbie and Johnnie did not like one another.

It was always interesting to watch the diver at work. My first memory of 'Johnnie the Diver' was large Pandrops. He always had a supply of these in his pocket and as they were about one and a half inches in diameter he had a novel way of reducing their bulk, which was even too big for an eager schoolboy's mouth. He wrapped the Pandrop in a red spotted hanky then smashed it with a claw hammer and retrieved the bits for me.

Johnnie later used the small grey hut between Lizzie's Tearoom and the weighbridge on the Esplanade in Lerwick as a diver's shed. All the diving apparatus was stored there and I spent many an hour watching him get ready. It was quite a performance and required the assistance of another man, usually the diver's linesman. I doubt if many of the present generation have seen the old type of diver or seen him being dressed so I will attempt to describe it as I remember it.

The diving suit was made of heavy canvas complete with feet, heavy rubber cuffs, and a rubber yoke attached to the suit, with holes in it at regular intervals front and back. These suits were normally stored on big wooden stretchers to dry them out. The diver first put on thick woollen drawers and cardigan. Then, sitting on a stool, he could slip his feet and legs into the suit before he stood up. After the diver had plunged his hands and wrists into a bucket of soft soap solution, the linesman could then pull the rubber cuffs over the diver's hands as far as the wrists. These cuffs were a very tight fit of necessity. At this stage the linesman had to pull and tug the heavy suit up over the diver's body, pulling out a canvas collar from within the yoke. Next, two metal plates, the shape of the yoke, with threaded studs had to be pulled below the rubber yoke and the studs passed through the holes. The breastplate was then passed over the diver's head and screwed down to these studs with wing nuts. Before, or at this stage, the diver's boots were laced on. They were very heavy and it took me all my time to lift one of them. If the diver had to walk a short distance to the ladder to descend into the sea his boots would be on but if the walk was more than a few yards the boots were laced on when he was nearer the ladder because of their immense weight. Next, a leather belt which had a knife in a sheath attached to it went round the middle. I thought it was for defence against sharks or giant octopuses, the influence of the picture house I expect.

Two very heavy lumps of lead in the shape of discs were lifted on to the front and back of the chest and attached with ropes to hang over the breast plate and were then tied round the diver's chest. A woolly hat was put on then the 'hard hat' or helmet lifted and lowered over the diver's head. The helmet was lowered, turned a quarter turn to the right then when engaged in the thread of the breast plate revolved a quarter turn to the left. This brought the round hole in the front of the helmet directly in front of the diver's face. The two airlines of reinforced rubber pipe were now tied down at the back to the breastplate. Lastly, the diver's lifeline, a strong, thin rope, was put on and tied via a lug on the helmet. When the diver had lumbered across to the ladder the linesman would guide his feet on to the first rung of the ladder, the diver facing the pier or vessel. Only then did the linesman screw in the glass face-plate, the pump men started pumping the air, the linesman gave the helmet a good smack as a final signal, and the diver descended. Once in the water he reached up to the valve on top of his helmet and regulated the escape of air to give him the required buoyancy. If he made a mistake he could shoot to the surface lying on his back looking like a 'Michelin man'. His arms would be spread-eagled, splinted by the suit so he could not reach up to his helmet to release more air. Thank goodness I never saw this happen, but was told it could with an inexperienced diver. Compared to modern self-contained diving suits, the old line diver was cumbersome in this suit and had his airlines dragging out behind him, limiting his mobility even further. He also had to take extra care when near any sharp object not to cut his airline. All signals in Johnnie's day were by tugs on the lifeline which the linesman paid out or took in slack as required on the edge of the pier, but holding the line taut enough to feel any signal from the diver.

My father learned to dive in the old suit, tutored by Johnnie. However, I don't think he enjoyed the experience too much and rarely did it.

Robbie Robertson, the other diver, had worked for my grandfather, J.W. Robertson, who formed the Scapa Flow Salvage and Shipbreaking Co. Ltd. in June, 1923. Though it was the firm of Cox and Danks which performed the difficult salvage of the German High Seas Fleet scuttled in Scapa Flow, the Shetland firm was the first to carry out salvage there on four destroyers. Robbie had dived on these and was later to dive on the *Oceanic* which J.W. had purchased from the Admiralty (for £200) as she lay on the Shaalds of Foula. He was dropped over the wreck from the Foula mailboat but found the tide so strong he could not keep his feet, let alone do any work, and had to be hurriedly pulled up. He refused to go down again and the salvage of some of the *Oceanic* had to wait until 1973 when modern diving gear enabled Simon Martin and Alec Crawford to recover some of the huge ship.

Robbie had many tall tales to tell and with no other diver having been near the *Oceanic* at that time, he could exaggerate his experiences without fear of contradiction. When diving at Scapa Flow he told one of his best whoppers. They had sailed, he said, from Lerwick in thick fog. It was so thick they could not even see the stem of the drifter and there was concern about sailing in these conditions, particularly the navigation. Robbie came up to the wheelhouse and belittled the problem by giving them a course to steer for a set period of time and then he was to be called. He then went below and turned in. His 'expertise' was called on at the stated time and he issued a further course change. This went on for some hours with frequent changes of course and the visibility remaining as before.

Eventually Robbie ordered, "Stop engines. Drop the hook when I tell you." Safely anchored, Robbie ordered his diving gear be brought up, got dressed and was lowered over the side, right down the funnel of the ship they were going to salve! Like all these stories, Robbie told them so often he believed them himself.

Whether Robbie was in the Navy in the first war or not, I don't know, but he told his best story of all with himself as the hero in the form of a Petty Officer.

Apparently Robbie was on a small boat which steamed round the Grand Fleet in Scapa with fresh water for the ships' boilers. There was a seaman on this vessel with him. One day, lying at the pier, Robbie had gone below to fix some engine problem, leaving the seaman on deck. *(The reader will realise that this was the first piece of ego building; Robbie being capable of engineering as well as everything else.)* Robbie, now suitably oily and greasy, was alerted by the seaman on deck who called down through the engine hatch, "Robbie, you had better come up for I see the Admiral's barge making for us."

Robbie said he was far too busy with the engine, and anyway, it would not be coming to them. The seaman became more and more agitated and excited so Robbie eventually went up on deck. Right enough, there was the Admiral's barge making straight for them. As he watched, they drew alongside with a great flurry of gold braid, bosun's pipe calls, twirling boathooks and as they tied up, an officer appeared from aft with gold tassels and things on his uniform, and jumped aboard their boat.

"Petty Officer Robertson?" he enquired.

"Yes sir, that's me," answered Robbie.

"You have to come with me immediately."

At this point Robbie said he would have to wash his hands and change out of his filthy boilersuit, but the officer said there was no time, just to come as he was. So, Robbie jumped aboard the Admiral's barge and they set off through the battleships and cruisers of the fleet. Eventually they were heading towards one particular battleship and Robbie realised that this was the *Iron Duke*, the flagship herself.

"Follow me," ordered the gold draped Lieutenant, so Robbie did as he was told: up the side of the battleship, salute the quarterdeck, through a steel door, along corridors, up more steps, through more steel doors and so on. *(Robbie made this journey last quite a considerable time when he told it.)*

Eventually, they reached a big steel door and stopped. The Lieutenant said, "Wait here," and he knocked and went in. In a second he was back, "Come inside, Robertson."

Robbie stepped into this huge room and as he came in, up jumped the Commander-in-Chief, Lord Jellicoe himself, and advanced on him with his hand out. "Thank God you've arrived, Robertson," the Admiral said, "the German fleet is out."

I lived for a short time in Scalloway and used to go up to Robbie's house. He had married a Foula woman and lived well up the hill in Scalloway. He made a model drifter for me which was a favourite toy. It had a wooden hull and a hold with a wooden hatch cover which could be lifted off. The wheelhouse was painted wood and the casing a tin tobacco box. The funnel was a piece of copper pipe, the capstan plus various other bits made from this and that. It looked very authentic, and was really rather good.

The last time I remember Robbie, he was standing on the fish market in Lerwick with a group of three or four men round him, laying off whilst the audience listened with grins on their faces. Robbie wore a black cheesecutter cap and he had a modern male hairstyle, in that his white hair was long and straggly, blowing all over the place in the wind. He reminded me of a broken down musician. One of the men speaking to him was my father and he came into the office afterwards laughing, to tell us the latest 'Robbie'. They had been discussing the award of an honour given to somebody locally in the birthday honours list. "OBE be damned!" Robbie exploded, "That's nothing."

"Why?" asked my father, "whit does du hae, Robbie?"

"I got the Croix de Guerre."

"Whar did du get it, Robbie?"

"I got it frae the Romanian government in the First World War."

My first teacher at the Central School was Miss Jamieson who lived at Baila at Sound. I note the house is still there almost unnoticed, as a simple white croft house in among the many new houses now in that area. She was a very good teacher, if lacking any sense of humour. It was work and work only and misdemeanours meant the strap. It was painful but had to be borne without flinching if you did not want to lose face. In fact it was essential to get the strap at some time to establish yourself with your male schoolmates. Miss Jamieson taught me the 'three Rs' thoroughly and I owe her a lot for the solid grounding which I received.

The next teacher was even more stern, and humourless, dedicated to teaching even the slowest of us and ruling with a rod of iron. One shout was sufficient to bring order even to the most unruly in the class. She was Mrs Bennet, a daughter of a previous headmaster, Durham, whom I believe was also a strict disciplinarian. (I was to be taught by another Durham later on and she was terrifying.)

In those days we went to school to learn and nothing else. It was not unpleasant, but it was not enjoyable and was jaundiced by continual anxiety over tests and examinations, particularly mental arithmetic, which was always terrifying. In retrospect, I realised how lucky I had been to have such an excellent teacher again in the important years leading up to the Control Examination.

And so, one Saturday morning I found myself at school to sit the Control Examination. I don't think I knew the significance of this test at the time but was told to sit it and did so. I passed and as a result moved after the summer holidays to a new school with new teachers and new subjects.

The bonus was increased greatly when a week or so later a knock at the door of the classroom revealed Alistair Fraser standing there. "Miss Garriock sent me up to you, sir, for..." (the three 'I' words were dutifully repeated).

"Well, well, Fraser, you do science don't you?"

"Yes, sir."

"You will come to my classroom for music periods in future. Go and sit there with Robertson."

Now Alistair was much better at science than I was and he was able to solve all sorts of problems in our homework for me.

This ended Alistair's and my musical education, but there was a sequel which illustrated so well A.T. Cluness' wisdom and understanding: a little later, again a knock at the door, this time Tom Black with the same tale from the music department.

"Do you like music, Black?"

A very emphatic, "No, sir!"

"Well, you will have another period a week of music to help you appreciate it."

Tom's face was a picture and we thoroughly enjoyed it. Poor Tom had to do his science homework after school and also had to suffer that awful class twice. Needless to say, there were no more knocks on the door.

Isn't it a pity we cannot appreciate some of the great things in life at that stage because we are too young and immature. Many years later I had an introduction to music in the smallest possible way and enjoyment of classical music grew from that: my father had a long playing record and one bit of it was very beautiful, this was the second movement of Mendelssohn's violin concerto and I repeatedly moved the stylus to play only that movement, graduating later to the whole piece. I regret that something in that style was not used in the school in those days.

I think back to Flora Campbell who tried to get us to appreciate the classics of English literature. She was so enthusiastic and therefore a good teacher. Part of the problem was that we had to read a chapter of the work under discussion at the time at home and then we went through it next day. Partly through the amount of homework and partly avoidance of anything we thought we might get away with, we rarely read the chapter previous to the class. The result was a much poorer understanding and appreciation of the classical novel. What pleasure I get today in comparison, but that is also because I have a lifetime of experience behind me. Poetry was another popular subject in English then and we learned to repeat lots of it in a parrot fashion. Later on, large passages from Shakespeare were learned and only superficially understood, in spite of good teachers like Lolly and John Graham in later classes. In recent years I have read and re-read most of the Shakespeare I did at school and have marvelled at how clever and discerning it is. Robert Burns is in the same category but was also difficult at school because of immaturity and the Scots tongue it was written in.

One English lesson I never forgot was a Shakespearean play – I think *Hamlet* – when the English teacher was absent. A.T. Cluness stood in and made the whole scene live by his explanation and obvious enthusiasm for the subject.

He showed he had a sense of humour right at the start of the class and immediately got our attention. "I remember," he said, "when I was doing *Hamlet* at school. The teacher asked us which character we would like to play. One boy answered 'Marshall Stock.' 'Marshall Stock,' said the teacher, 'I can't recall him in Hamlet.' 'Oh yes, sir,' the pupil insisted, 'he's in it.' 'Show me where in the play you saw him.' 'There,' said the pupil, 'Hamlet enters with *martial stalk*.' "

Art and I might have got along very well, and I say that now in the light of what it became in my life, but the teacher and I never did get along. The art teacher in those days was Dorothy Johnson. She again did not seem to have any sense of humour and worse still there was a rigid course to be followed and no possibility of self expression, something which has become an excuse today for anything in so-called art. As a result of this clash of personalities, the subject was suffered but not enjoyed or taken seriously. When I consider now how lucky I was to have an evening class teacher in art twenty years later at Baltasound, who gradually extracted any little talent I had and changed the whole world around me, perhaps it was just as well that I did not appreciate the narrow discipline of the art class at school.

Things came to a bit of a pitch one day in the art room. We sat at painting desks on stools with a seat which sloped forwards. There was always a bit of necessary movement to the sink for water and I was seen by Dorothy tipping a little water on to the back of one or two stools as I came back from the sink. This water ran down the stool but it took a few seconds for the water to penetrate the appropriate trousers or skirt. By the time the pupil jumped up grabbing his wet bum I was safely back in my seat busily engaged in my work. I did not know I had been seen until a large book thudded down on top of my head and she said, "Bobby, you are a nincompoop!" There were sniggers all round and that made me snigger too so I was sent outside the door for the rest of the period. Now the art room door opened directly into the hall and this banishment suited me fine as the girls were doing physical education in the hall in their knickers.

During my time at the Institute one of my pals was Arthur Laurenson, later to succeed his father as Clerk to the Lerwick Harbour Trust. Arthur had a Shetland model boat and I had my first introduction to sailing with him. We rigged up an old tent on an oar and sailed before the wind up Leiraness Voe in Bressay. We then had to row out the voe into the wind and repeat the procedure. Not only that, the only way the boat seemed to sail with this pathetic rig was with a list so we both lay on one side of the boat and, being so near the water, it appeared to us we were flying.

Later I got the loan of a four-oared yoal. This was a super boat to row and had a mast step for a lug sail. Tammy Anderson from Whalsay had moved down to Burns Lane and he was a great companion in a boat. Most of what I learned about boats was due to him and it was only when I acquired a small lug sail that Tammy became less keen. The fact of the matter was that I was very keen but inexperienced and Tammy was more experienced and wiser.

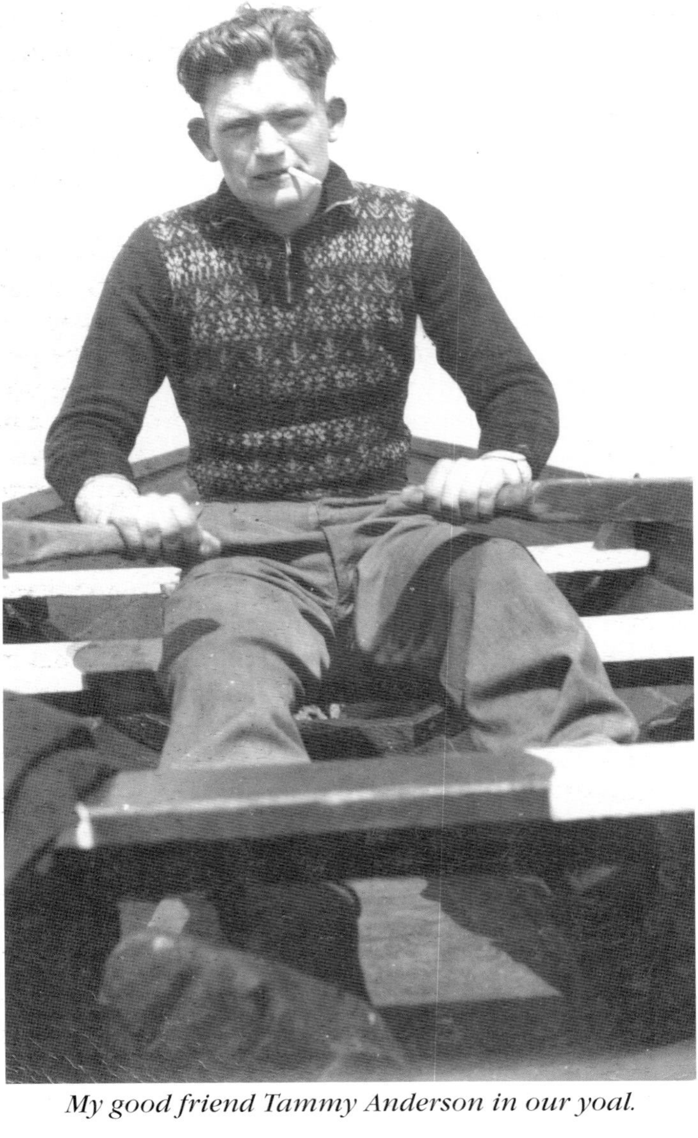

My good friend Tammy Anderson in our yoal.

Mostly we just rowed. This caused a great deal of anxiety one day when we decided to go to Start Point at the north end of Bressay to fish for olicks. It took us about an hour and a half to row there and we fished rather unsuccessfully for a couple of hours before starting to row back. The wind had freshened from the west and probably we had tide against us as well because it was well after tea time by the time we arrived back. I lived by this time at the South End in Lerwick and we were met with a stormy reception. We resented the reaction, not then aware of the worry we had caused.

Tammy had got a new 'tully' of which he was immensely proud and one evening off the Bressay light he reluctantly allowed Spud Thomson to borrow it for cutting up some bait. He was gutting some herring on a board and throwing the guts over the starboard side but busy talking at the same time. Spud threw the next lot over the port side, and was left sitting with a handful of guts! I thought Tammy was going to murder Spud there and then, but he was really a gentle giant and had enough sense not to start that sort of thing in a boat.

On another occasion herring had come right up to the Knab so we got an old herring net and went off with it one evening. Have you ever tried to work with a herring net in a yoal? It was difficult to get the cork upper end sorted out in the boat, the net caught in every rough edge of wood, let alone buttons and the other snags in the boat. We did eventually get it in the water but without a bush rope it lay in a bundle and would not form a vertical curtain. We caught no herring.

Later at school I became friendly with Tom and Jim Black from Quendale and, along with Bobby Johnson and Arthur Laurenson, I spent many weekends at Brake. Tom introduced me to the .22 rifle and we had expeditions to Fitful Head. There was a reasonably easy route to the bottom of the cliffs at one spot and plenty of seals there. The idea was to creep down unseen and to shoot a seal on the shore. If we shot one further out we could not retrieve it. We did get one and flayed it there and then so that we could carry the skin back. What we smelled like with all the blubber and oil I hate to think, let alone what oil seeped into our clothes as we carried the skin back over our shoulders. We sold it for 10 shillings to a man, Angus, out the North Road.

It is said school days are the happiest days of your life and to some extent my experiences at the Institute agreed with this. There did not seem to be any goal but things just rolled along from one weekend to the next. It always seemed to be a bit of a struggle to get all the homework done at a weekend. I never felt entirely relaxed until it was out of the way. I found a fixed pattern was best and I started immediately on arrival home from school on Friday afternoon. Later that evening I had broken the back of it. Little did I know what was to come; what I spent in minutes then would not compare to the hours spent later.

However, all good things come to an end and the Highers were about to be tackled. It was only then that I discovered that things did not look too rosy. Everybody just went to school, sat and passed examinations or had to leave, or drop back to repeat a year and at the end of it all pass some further examinations and go on to university. It was a fixed path with no diversions, not that anybody questioned the route. Firstly it was decided that I would probably not get Higher French, so I would have to sit the Lower. I must say that I tended to agree with that opinion. However, it was decided that I was doubtful for Higher Science and would be better to sit the Lower. Not only did this rob me of a university entrance but it meant part of the paper was in biology which I had not done much of previously and then only in the junior classes.

There was no career advice, nor indeed any advice of any kind. What would look better on the overall school results appears to have been paramount. My parents were not academics so could not advise me or perhaps insist I had the chance to sit enough for a university entrance.

So, at eighteen, I had higher maths and English, and lower French, science and history. Three highers and two lowers was the minimum university entrance requirement. At the end of class six I left school and it was only then that I began to realise that I was qualified for nothing.

Chapter 3

Out in the world

THE realisation that I would now have to try and make my way in the world and earn my keep with minimum qualifications to do so, gradually became more of a worry and I was willing to do anything, rather like Mr Micawber, hoping something would turn up. Of course, this was a very optimistic view which could only have been held by an eighteen year old. I got various short jobs, one of which was a clerk in the local National Insurance office. This was boring to say the least and I think did a lot to jolt me into some sort of decision.

I would at some time have to do two years national service so volunteered for early call-up and asked for the RAF. Within two weeks I had my call-up papers to report to RAF Padgate on 1st November, 1950.

The journey down to Aberdeen by the *St Clair II*, then train to Edinburgh, took most of a day and I had some hours in Edinburgh before catching another train about 10 o'clock that night. I was fortunate to have a cousin in the city and was well looked after and then taken to the train. The journey seemed interminable, partly because it was cold and dark and unknown, but eventually I arrived at Warrington in Lancashire at 6am on a dark, rainy, miserable November morning. Warrington was a grim, industrial town which would not have looked inviting even in mid summer. A bus was waiting at the station and a number of us were transported to Padgate and a new life.

That introduction will always remain in my mind as the worst breakfast I had ever seen. An empty mess hall which seemed to be huge, a row of mess orderlies behind a counter, a plate onto which went a splash of wet material that turned out to be mashed potato, some material which vaguely resembled bacon, a slice of bread with margarine, and instructions to help ourselves to tea. The tea came out of urns in the middle of the floor, either sugary or not, and I at that time took sugar so filled a mug. It was a greyish colour with a strange smell and the first mouthful made me wonder how I was going to drink this stuff for two years. This was merely a receiving camp for the thousands of national servicemen that poured through here each month and it was amazing how quickly the awfulness of this food diminished so that at the end of a week I could manage to eat and drink enough to survive. Fortunately there was a NAAFI canteen where a fry-up and slightly better tea could be purchased in the evening.

We were kitted out, boots to cap, and all was shoved into a kit bag along with a tangled lot of webbing, small pack, large pack and water bottle, mug, knife, fork and spoon. Everybody got a number and this was stamped on the kit bag. We attended lectures, stood in long single files then walked in a door where a needle was jabbed in your arm and out a door on the other side. Nobody explained what these injections were, but they certainly had immunisation down to a rapid fine art. Every hour we were marched to another venue and time went quickly.

At the end of a week, small groups of us had become friends only to be broken up as we were transported to the railway station and put on board various trains. Nobody knew where or why we were moving and strangely nobody seemed to ask; it was accepted as the next part of the adventure.

I was in a crowd which did not have to travel very far before we arrived at a pretty little station called Wilmslow in Cheshire. Our kit was put in a lorry and we marched, after a fashion, up a steep hill. We were told that when we left we would carry our kit to the station as we would be different men by the end of the next eight weeks. It sounded a bit ominous and proved to be very accurate. On arrival in an open hangar at RAF Wilmslow the kit bags were thrown out of the lorry and the last three numbers shouted out for each. You had to run and collect your kit and then run back in line. My last three was '901' and this label preceded your surname at all times if you were addressed directly. Pay parade each week required a smart step forward, a salute at "901", all for one pound. We then went to our billets which were wooden huts round a huge tarmac square.

On arrival at the billet we were amazed at the shine on the linoleum floor and wondered what all the felt pads were at the door as we came in. This wonder did not last long for a corporal appeared, not very tall but with beret pulled right down over one eye, webbing belt and gaiters and a short stick under his arm. "My name is Wimpenny and I am God here. As soon as I or any other NCO appears the first man to see him will jump to attention and shout NCO. Everybody drops what they are doing and stands to attention at the foot of his bed. Now, you see this floor?"

"Yes, corporal," we answered.

"Shining, isn't it?"

A very emphatic, "Yes, corporal," was the universal reply.

"Well, it's shitty to what it is going to be by 10 o'clock tonight."

He then went round the hut, running his finger along ledges, etc. and finding layers of dust which we had not noticed. He looked inside the two bogey stoves in the hut and said they were disgusting as indeed were the outsides of the stove. The hearthstones were whitewashed and the insides of the coal buckets, to my surprise, were also white. Numerous other faults in the cleanliness were discovered until I began to have difficulty in keeping tally of what we had to do to satisfy this martinet by ten o'clock that night. Various cleaning materials were produced. Big bumpers were used for polishing the floor. We were informed we must never walk on the floor but shuffle about on two of the felt pads at the door. This of course helped a lot over the weeks to keep this mirror surface the way it had to be. There was some flurry of activity when he left and we were in the middle of this when "NCO" rang out from near the ablution door, which was at the other end of the hut leading down a short passage to the toilets, showers and wash-hand basins.

At the time it was very funny and to this day I still smile when I think about it: at the door stood a flight sergeant of RAF police complete with white gaiters, white webbing belt, white cheesecutter cap pulled right down to eye level, and this frightening man was flanked by two corporals similarly kitted out. We stood at attention in two lines at the foot of the two rows of beds for perhaps a minute but it seemed much longer and not a word was spoken.

When this tyrant spoke he had used the long silence to good effect as his great authority was obvious to us all. "Children," he said, and then a long pause while we stared at the man opposite, scared to blink an eye. "Children," he then said again, "yes, all recruits are children to me. Now children, when you go to bed tonight you will put your wallet underneath your pillow. Understand?"

"Yes, flight sergeant," we chorused.

"I don't want any children coming down to the guard room and saying, 'Please, flight sergeant, I have lost my wallet.' Is that clear?"

Yet again there was a solid chorus from the children.

"Any questions?" he asked.

Nobody said anything for a moment. Directly across the room, opposite to me, there was a round, freckly-faced fellow with sandy colouring who always seemed to have a half smile on his face. His name was Rooney and he came from Liverpool. He stuck up his hand.

"Yes, what is it?" the flight sergeant asked.

"Please, flight sergeant, what do you do with your small change?"

I have never felt so ill in my life; to have to stand at attention without a flicker of expression on your face under these circumstances was almost too much to bear. I longed to double up and it was worse because so many others were suffering the same agony of suppression. To make it even worse, the flight sergeant stood absolutely still and said nothing for a long while, then said, "Have you ever had your arse kicked, laddie?"

"No, flight sergeant," Rooney replied.

"Well, you're bloody well asking for it!" And with that they wheeled around and left the billet. The entire 31 of us collapsed immediately, except Rooney who did not see what we were all laughing at.

It was November or December and deep snow. The cold in the billet was intense as we could not light the two bogey stoves as there was not time in the morning to wash, shave, dress, make up the mathematically correct biscuit of sheets and blankets on the bed, arrange various items, e.g. razor, etc, on the bedside shelf (also in mathematical order), clean the various ledges under the bed and elsewhere, polish the floor if any marks were apparent, and appear at seven o'clock in darkness and snow to be marched up to the cookhouse for what they called 'breakfast', as well as to blacken two stoves, whiten the coal buckets inside, polished outside, and whiten the hearthstones as well as clean out the fire and clean the inside of the stove.

As a result our boots were frozen to the floor in the morning and my mug with water, which I took to bed with me, was frozen solid in the morning. Shetlanders may have to suffer chill factors well below freezing due to winter wind, but never did I experience such intense cold air frost as in Cheshire that winter. Rooney sent home for a hot water bottle - a forbidden item. He filled it out of the hot water tap in the ablutions and after five minutes at his feet in bed he passed it on to his neighbour who had a few minutes and passed it on until it reached number 32, i.e. back to Rooney. I may say it was not very hot to begin with but it was only tepid by number 31, but even that was heavenly.

It really felt like being a prisoner; up at 6am, all this panic to clean and be clean, the march to the cookhouse at 7am with one arm holding knife, fork, spoon and mug in the small of the back, march back, having dipped these utensils in the big tank of boiling dirty water at the door as you came out.

Rooney caused more mirth quite innocently later when he got muddled up with RAF terms and answered, "Yes, squadron," to the corporal. I can't remember the insults he suffered nose to nose with Corporal Wimpenny. Throughout square-bashing there was a great camaraderie in the billet. If someone got some punishment or 'jankers', everybody rallied round to help him clean his kit, blanco his webbing, small and large pack, press his trousers, polish his boots or whatever: comradeship in adversity. Unfortunately, after we left there I never saw it again to the same extent.

The chap in the next bed to me came from rural Devon; a farmer's son and a real yokel. The name of the farm was Woolfarthersworthy and he was so much the simple country lad that eventually the NCOs had to admit defeat. They always addressed him as "Woolfarthersworthy" and he had a rough passage to begin with, but they were human enough to see the impossibility of turning him into a 'guardsman' and seemed to accept him for the helpless recruit he was. When it came to the pinnacle of the eight weeks square-bashing, Woolfarthersworthy was detailed as barrack orderly to avoid him disrupting the passing out parade.

I was sent for a haircut one day and you had to report to the station warrant officer after it was done. I seem to remember his name was Tudor. Anyway, he asked me where I came from and when I said Shetland he became quite human and said he had been at Sullom Voe during the war. This was just before Christmas and he asked me if I was going home on Xmas leave. I said I would rather have gone home for New Year. The result was that I was put on fire piquet over Christmas and got my leave at New Year. I also missed a few days of square-bashing as a result.

We were very fortunate to have a nice sergeant. He shouted and barked like the rest but was a bit more human than the corporals. We had, by this time, learned never to volunteer for anything however pleasant it was purported to be. One day on parade, Sgt Thorley asked for two baby-sitters. I stuck up my hand and was very relieved to discover that it was genuine for a change. "Report to the guardroom you two at 7pm." We did so and were allowed outside the camp for the first and only time in the eight weeks, though I did manage to get out once more, but to that later. What a bonus the baby-sitting proved to be. We were shown Sgt Thorley's kitchen with bacon, eggs, sausages, etc., and told to make ourselves some supper. What a marvellous meal we had and the children slept through so we were not really needed. At about midnight the sergeant and his wife came home and we went back to camp. We had some difficulty at the guardroom avoiding arrest for being absent without leave, but a phone call to the sergeant sorted it out for us.

Our difficulties of admission to the camp always brought to mind a story I heard about two WAAFs who were too late and decided to crawl under the barbed wire. As they were doing this, one said to the other, "I feel like a commando."

"So do I," reflected the other, "but where do you think we would find two at this time of night?"

One Sunday I was told to report to the guardroom. This was normally bad news as whatever the business at the guardroom you might consider yourself lucky to get away again without being put on a charge for some trivia of dress, or anything the policeman on duty contrived to find if he was in that mood.

But when I got there, who was sitting there but an old grand aunt from the Burgh Road in Lerwick. "We have come to take you out for your tea in Manchester."

I could not get her to understand that I was not allowed out of the camp, but she was a bit of a madam in her own way and she somehow beat them down to a short pass. Her son lived in Manchester and she was visiting. It was very kind and considerate and I enjoyed the freedom for an afternoon. The only thing I can remember about it was on the journey back to Manchester. Auntie Maggie said she would need the ladies'. Her son said, "Well, the only one is 'The Green Lion'."

"Is that a public house?" she asked.

"Yes," he replied.

"I would rather be seen dead than to enter a public house," she said.

However, she had to enter the gates of hell when her bladder could not withstand the pressure any longer. I was amused to smell alcohol on her son's breath when he came out to the car with her afterwards.

Examinations again appeared but they were very basic, simple questions and I found I was eligible for a Group B trade as a result. Group A was the best, but only available for regular airmen, not national servicemen.

My choice was between armourer and wireless technician as far as I can recall. Not much of a choice but a great relief not to be allocated kitchen work or something as boring. I had, like everyone else, spent days on fatigues, digging coal, sweeping up parade grounds or hangars, being a general factotum in the cookhouse or worse still, delegated to the 'tin room'. I remember one day spent there where all the huge cooking tins and utensils arrived for washing in a very hot tank with something like washing soda in the water. No gloves or refinements meant very sore hands and it was also wet and unpleasant. Peeling potatoes was much more preferable.

At the end of square-bashing it had all become reasonably routine. The pressure from the NCOs decreased as we approached the end and, of course, we had a final night in the NAAFI which the NCOs attended. Looking back, it must have been an awful bore for them but they became human beings after all that final night.

My posting was to RAF Kirkham, just outside Blackpool, for trade training which lasted three months, nearly all spent in classrooms and workshops. There were three categories of armourer – turrets, guns or bombs. I was allocated bombs and for the next twelve weeks worked on every type of bomb then available, from the 23,000lb armour piercing to practice bombs weighing 12lb and 25lb. It was interesting to see the 23,000lb bomb, called the Tall Boy, which was used to attack U-boat pens,

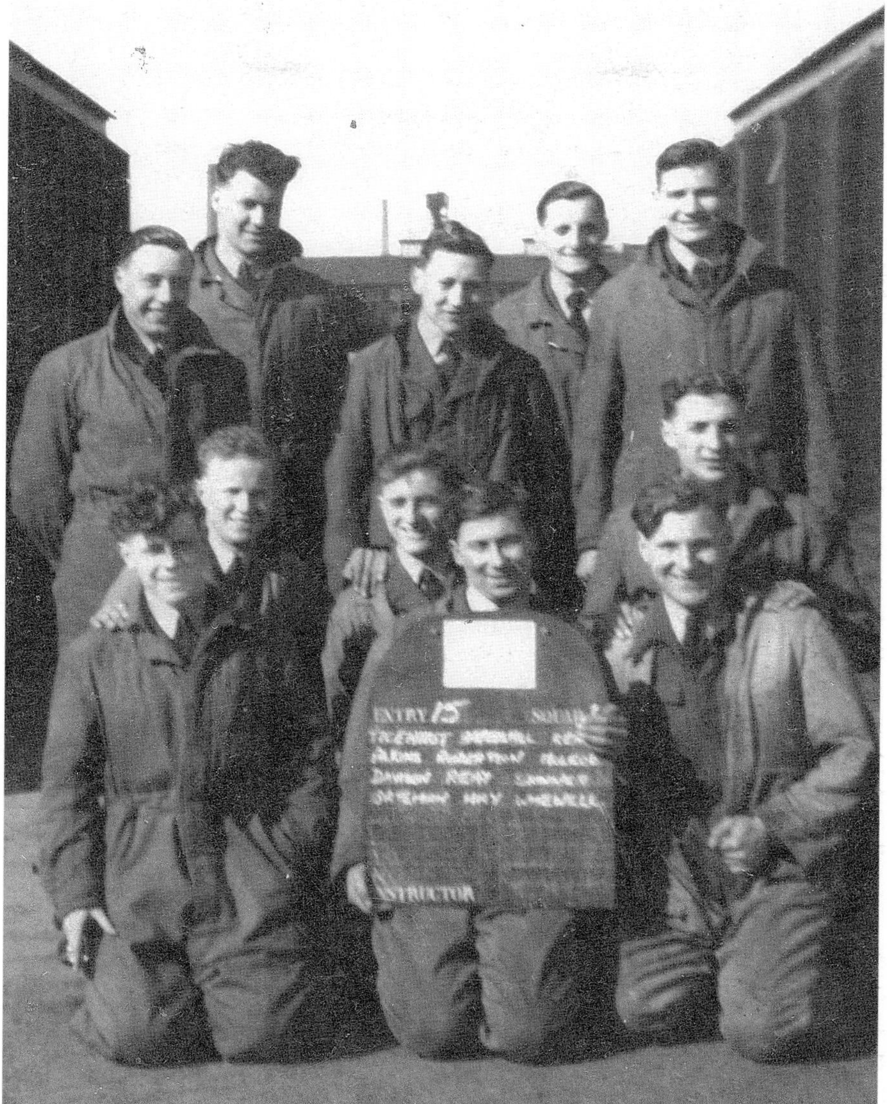

Armourer trade training at RAF Kirkham, Lancs., in 1951 (the author is middle, standing).

the *Tirpitz* in Norway, and targets of that sort. The 12,000lb non-penetrating bomb consisted of three large barrels bolted together, each of 4,000lb. We examined German bombs and did a course on aerial depth charges, pyrotechnics of all sorts and many bomb pistols, including various delay mechanisms. Examinations took place regularly and there was a fair amount to assimilate and then regurgitate at the exams.

We were now allowed weekends free so went into Blackpool, but it was completely commercial and I hated it. We earned £1 a week and to get a NAAFI supper and buy cigarettes took half of it at least, so a cream bun and a cup of tea and later a fish supper was about all we could get in Blackpool.

I went to Liverpool with one of my fellow armourers one weekend. We went to a bridge alongside the Grand National course to watch the race which was running that particular Saturday. I could see nothing the first time the horses went by, but did manage to clamber up some railings to see one or two riderless horses pass by, followed by a half a dozen with riders. It all lasted about a minute and needless to say that was the end of my race going. I never could see the attraction except for the gambling, which for us on £1 a week was not an option.

I passed my trade test and awaited my posting, hoping to be sent somewhere nearer home. Eventually the postings were put up on the notice board. Everybody was posted to within two or three hours at most from home. My posting was to RAF Gosport, across from Portsmouth, about as far from Shetland as was possible. Two other armourers were also posted to Gosport, both from London. However, at least it meant company from Kirkham and a guide through the Underground in London for me. I had, up until that time, never seen the tube, let alone found my way from one railway station to another by means of it.

We arrived in London about 4.30pm and once on the tube had to transfer to get to the Portsmouth train. It was very hot, terribly crowded and, of course, with all our kit and a kitbag on top of the large pack across your shoulders it was not easy to make your way through. It meant also that your head was bent forwards and you looked more or less at your feet, with occasional glances upwards. I explain this because of one of those coincidences which is almost unbelievable.

We got through this huge throng of hurrying people at that time of the evening rush-hour, arrived on the train platform and thankfully dumped our kit bags off our shoulders. I had just done so when I felt a tap on the shoulder. I looked round and there was Elsie Craigie from Unst, who had gone through the Institute with me. She'd thought it was me going up a moving staircase as she came down on the other side. It was very observant of her as my attitude, as I have said, did not give a clear view of my face, and the uniform was strange to her. Anyway, she lived with an aunt in Victoria Street so that was a home from home if I should ever need it. I did spend one day later on my way home on leave with Elsie, but I have never seen her since.

Chapter 4

Armourer mechanic (bombs)

RAF Fort Grange was a strange RAF station. In fact it could not have been stranger. We had to get off the train at its terminus, I think it was Portsmouth Harbour, and then take a small ferry across the harbour to a Royal Navy camp at Gosport called, like all navy camps, HMS something or other. Across a road, and a hundred yards or so further up the road lay Fort Grange, built in the shape of a hollow circle with a large arched entrance. The fort had been built in the Napoleonic era during the invasion scare of the time. The circular wall was about forty feet in height and at least that in thickness, completely overgrown on top. Inside the walls of the fort lay the square, some wooden huts which formed the cookhouse, and the motor transport section. Apart from a guardroom in a hut at the gate, I can't remember much else. However, all round the walls were semi-circular tunnels built into the walls and these were the billets. At the rear of the billets there was a dark stone corridor that connected the billets to the ablutions. These consisted of galvanised trays with a tap at the end of each which had a short length of rubber hose attached to it. It was all very primitive and the billets had whitewashed stone curved ceilings. These must have been terrible places to live in the winter but it was now May and very hot, so the billets were pleasurably cool. It was so hot that I found it impossible to sit out in the sun.

Not only was the camp unusual in this way, but the work situation was even stranger. There was an aerodrome up behind the fort at a higher level but it was a Royal Naval air station and we, the armourers, appeared to be some of the few RAF among all the sailors. Furthermore, the only armament for the planes was torpedoes and the navy had a workshop where these were maintained. None of us had done torpedoes as part of our course so we sat about all day from eight to five reading papers or any other thing to pass the time. It was crazy and I very quickly got fed up with nothing to do.

After a few weeks of this idleness, I decided to apply for my first ever normal leave. I managed to get two days travelling time each way and a week's leave. I needed the travelling time as it took most of the two days to get by train to London, then to Aberdeen and thence by steamer to Lerwick.

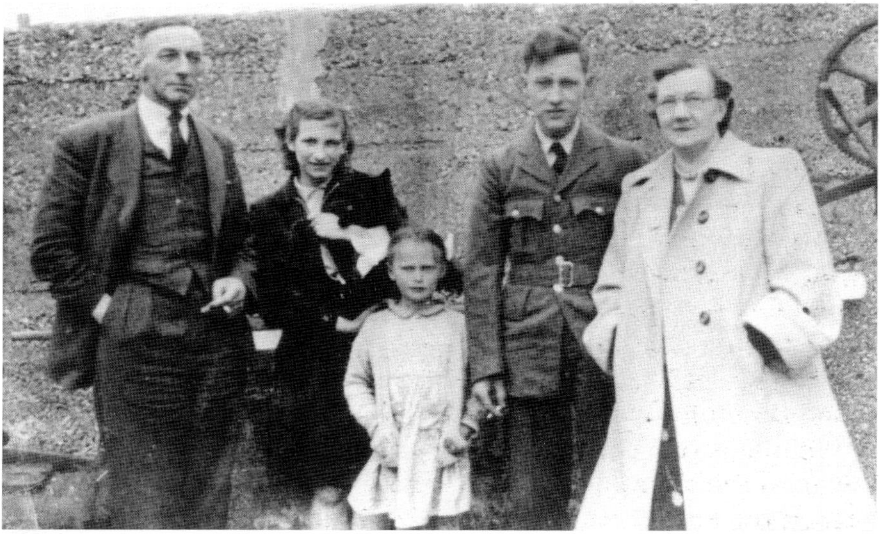

With father, sister Mona, sister Joan and mother at No.12 Commercial Street.

When I went to the orderly room to get my pass with the rail warrants, a sergeant called Ross, a Scot, said, "You're a long way from home."

"Just about as far as I can get," I replied.

"I will see what I can do for you. Come and see me when you come back from leave."

Off I went, but had difficulty in holding on to some of the travel warrant as it said Portsmouth to Lerwick. The railway ticket collector wanted to keep the travel warrant but I required the whole document to get my steamer ticket. However, they eventually, reluctantly, allowed me to keep the papers.

When I came back after two days travelling again, I went to see Sgt Ross and he said, "Pack your bags, you're posted to Kinloss."

I have never forgotten that kindness and still remember that sergeant who was so considerate. I don't know how he did it. Probably he had a pal in 'movements' who could arrange postings. I promptly cleared the fort and two days later I was back in Aberdeen on my way to Forres and RAF Kinloss.

Kinloss was a busy air station and belonged to RAF Coastal Command. There were two parts to it: a squadron which was independent of the rest and an air conversion side where pilots learned how to fly four-engined aircraft after two-engined planes. I was on this operation conversion unit as an armourer mechanic bombs. The planes were Lancasters which had been in the war and were rapidly becoming obsolete. After a few months these were phased out and we got Avro Shackletons.

The Lancasters were interesting to work on but loading bombs, usually just practice bombs, could be hazardous. The electrics were unreliable and I have seen practice bombs fall off the bomb racks because of electrical faults. The height from the front of a Lancaster bomb bay was about 20 feet. We also loaded depth charges but these were 250lb and had to be winched up into the bomb bay. The Shackletons were much roomier to work inside and the bomb bay not so high.

I eventually rose to the dizzy heights of senior aircraftsman and could go no further as a national serviceman. It was in this capacity that I became the senior armourer of a party of three who did night duty. On one particular night it was the Lancasters which had to be 'bombed up' with depth charges for a certain take-off time. I was the only one of the three licensed to drive the tractor and therefore had to fetch the depth charges from the bomb dump a few miles away. This was done and I set the two armourers to load the charges. Some of the bomb racks failed to show lights on testing and had to be changed so there was a delay in 'take-off' time. The two lads on with me were new and did not know much about the job. Anyway, about 2am the Lancasters came back but had not dropped their charges, so we had to lower them all down by winch back on to the bomb trolleys. During this, the tractor went on fire and it was decided, after I got it out, to offload the charges and do two or three runs back to the bomb dump. I wrote my report and went back to the billet at 8am to get some sleep.

Shortly afterwards I was wakened and told to come down to the armament section at the aerodrome. I was met by the warrant officer, who was second-in-command in the armament section, and asked for an explanation for the delay in take-off and why I had left half a dozen depth charges lying on the grass in front of the wing commander's window. I thought I had explained everything in the night flying report, but not so. The warrant officer was a very nice man and he then went in to report to the section officer. I would have to report to the boss, he told me when he came out. I really expected to be on a charge now and was very lucky to get a severe ticking off from this officer. W.O. Sheed I think saved my bacon. I had simply forgotten the depth charges in among the stress of burning tractors and pressure to unarm all three aircraft at once. The flight sergeant was also a decent man and it was a happy section to work in.

One of our armourers who was a junior technician, that is a much more highly trained man who had done an apprenticeship in the RAF and was on a 12-year contract, was not so lucky. He left a 20mm cannon shell live in one of the cannons in a Shackleton after gun practice. He got seven days jankers but he had been in the service for a few years and it did not seem to put him up or down.

The camaraderie at this stage was only among a small group of friends, not general as it had been in the days of 'adversity'. I cannot remember anybody offering to clean his brasses or blanco his webbing and packs or polish his boots. These were inspected at every hourly visit to the guardroom in full kit. These visits started early in the morning before work, then resumed after work until 10pm. If any bit of kit did not come up to scratch a further few days' punishment could be added.

Unfortunately there were too many armourers for the work available and it had become the clever thing to 'skive' at work. We had a crew room in the section which consisted of a small room with our wooden tool boxes set along each wall. This formed the seating. The only other furnishing consisted of coat hooks which were for overalls. It had a radiator and, although simple and basic, it seemed to be almost like a club room at the time. The routine was to turn up for work at 8am. Shortly after eight the sergeant would come into the crew room and allocate jobs. This was the time to be absent and hope you were overlooked. A few of us did the *Daily Express* crossword each day and there was some competition to be the first to finish. This passed the time for an hour or so bringing us up to NAAFI break about 10am. I became quite good at 'skiving' like everybody else but soon realised that it was a much longer day sitting about on a box than working so made sure I was allocated a task. I even volunteered to weed the flower beds in front of the section just to have something to do. Later on I found this attitude probably helped me when I applied for a special three-day pass to sit examinations in Aberdeen. The pass was issued without even an interview – a rather rare event.

We all had calendars with the days marked off until demob. The catch phrase for national servicemen was "Roll on death, demob is too slow". It was in this billet that I first became aware of Catholic/Protestant hatred, particularly among the Glasgow airmen. They hurled abuse at one another in the billet at night and it became very tedious. However, I never actually saw any physical violence. I had been naive as regards religious divides until then. I was also quite intrigued by the fact that a man in the next bed was a Jew. I had never been aware of them before apart from the one shopkeeper in Lerwick. I did not, of course, recognise this airman as a Jew until it was pointed out to me by the more worldly wise of my colleagues.

Air training cadets were sometimes seen at the weekend at Kinloss and one day one of these young boys was caught smoking a cigarette under the wing of a Shackleton in a hangar by one of the hangar sergeants. If I remember correctly, the wing above his head held about 1,600 gallons of petrol. "Put that cigarette out!" bawled the sergeant, whereupon the cadet said, "But I'm old enough to smoke, sergeant."

In these pre-TV times the main source of recreation in the evenings seemed to be cards. This was harmless but the gambling

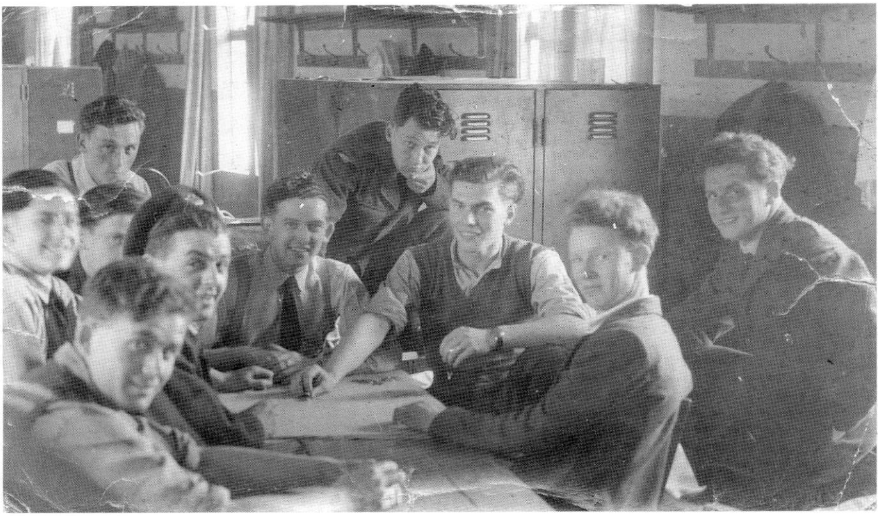

A game of cards, with stakes, in the billet at RAF Kinloss (the author is watching at the back).

element took over. Brag and poker attracted a big crowd in the billet. It was a disaster for some, especially on pay night, who lost all then had to borrow, if he could, for the coming week. This, of course, meant he started off the next week broke again. It never did attract me and though I often watched, I never played.

The later part of my time was taken up with a course in the evenings, but what I did before I can't remember. We always went out in a group on Saturday afternoons and went to a dance somewhere on Saturday night. Eventually we discovered the best place was Keith in Banffshire. It took about half an hour to get there by train and there was a Commercial Hotel in Mid Street which gave us a cheap rate for bed & breakfast on Saturday night and Sunday morning. There was a local dance and we always ended up there. We did not like Inverness or Elgin, and Forres was overcrowded.

One of our Shackletons had been forced to land in Lincolnshire at RAF Waddington. When it was airworthy volunteers were requested to fly down in another Shackleton with the relief crew and, when we had done an inspection on the stranded aircraft, fly back in it. An armourer was required as it had depth charges in the bomb bay and they had to be checked and rendered safe before take-off. The only snag was it was a weekend, but I considered it worth it to get a chance to fly in a Shackleton. There was an added bonus of a night in Lincoln, the one and only time I have been there. The trip back was a treat on the Sunday morning due to lovely weather and the pilot flew along the coast of England and then Scotland before diverting across to Kinloss. It was interesting to see the map which I knew so well from school laid out below. I spent most of the time in the mid upper gun turret as it afforded a complete all round view and, anyway, it was part of my province. The seat was comfortable and by means of a joystick the whole turret could be revolved in any direction you chose.

Apart from the odd diversion like this, the posting was pretty routine and like most jobs, apart from a few parades and the military discipline.

When we had Lancasters at Kinloss they were capable of carrying an airborne lifeboat. This boat was carried outside the belly under the bomb bay with the doors closed. It was our job to hoist it up and fix it in position. If required, it was released from a special hook which extruded through the bomb bay doors. Three parachutes took it down to the sea and when it hit the water they were automatically released and, at the same time, a rocket from each side fired out a light orange cotton line at right angles, to aid the survivors getting hold of the lifeboat. From the bow a line with a sea anchor was shot out thus to slow the lifeboat's drift and help keep her head to wind.

I acquired one of these rocket lines at the end of its useful life and found it an excellent hand-line. I always seemed to catch more fish than anybody else in the boat and decided that it must be the luminosity of the orange colour that attracted the fish. I remember discussing this with Dr Peter Peterson and he was firmly convinced that a light at the end of a hand-line would attract fish. The problem of waterproofing the torch he thought might be solved by means of a condom! My line lasted a few years but being cotton it eventually rotted and I never had the same success with other lines.

Every time the Queen flew up to Balmoral we had to put an airborne lifeboat up on a Lancaster. When she arrived at Dyce we had to take it down again. Her Majesty was not too popular when she flew at weekends, and I could never understand the need when the flight path from London to Aberdeen was entirely over land.

After I had been a year in the RAF I began to consider my future again. I decided to try the prelims at Aberdeen University in physics and chemistry, if I could study sufficiently. After all, I had done the course at school, and if I could pass it would give me a university entrance. The RAF, to give it its due, was always prepared to help anybody study and I went up to the Education Department to enquire about help to study by means of a correspondence course. Again I was lucky because the second-in-command of this section turned out to be Ian Fraser, who had been at school with me, although a few years ahead of me. He now had a degree and as such was an education officer. This not only made it easy for me to speak to him, but naturally he was a great help and managed to get me the required correspondence course.

Now I had my hands full, work during the day and a course to complete and send off each week. There was no hope of any study in the billet but I discovered the writing room in the NAAFI which was little used and so spent all my evenings during the week doing physics and chemistry.

The next step was to apply for one extra day off as the physics examination was at Aberdeen University on a Saturday, which was suitable, but the chemistry was on Monday. I had an aunt in Aberdeen so accommodation was no problem and, as I have said, I had good bosses at Kinloss, so it was easily arranged.

I sat both and quite honestly did not have any idea how I had done. A telegram from home some weeks later simply said, "Pass in physics, pass in chemistry." After that I often wondered whether I might have been saved all the hassle and, indeed, if I had had enough passes to go to university I would then have had an easier time in the services as a medical officer after graduation. It's like the dentist, nice when you come out and also satisfying to know you have done what you know you had to do. My national service was like that and I never really regretted doing it the way I did as it gave me two extra years to mature before starting university. So often I saw students of 17 or 18 who got carried away with the social life at university and were not mature enough to realise their future was at stake.

Now I had a problem which might prove to be insurmountable. The university term started in October and here I was in the RAF, not due for demobilisation until the 7th November. First I had to decide which faculty to apply for, then submit an application and only on acceptance of that could I start an application to the service asking for a premature discharge. I thought at the time that it was unlikely they would let me off with part of my two years. In that case I might have to wait another year before starting.

I started to eliminate the courses I did not want to do and also those which were not suitable for me. Divinity was easily discarded for a start. Arts appeared to be too airy fairy for me and I wanted something more physically active than law. This left me with science, dentistry or medicine. I had spoken to John H. Spence, the Director of Education in Shetland at that time, when I was doing the correspondence course and he tried hard to convince me that I would make more money in dentistry than any of the others. I was not convinced and, after the struggle to get higher chemistry and physics, science did not seem to be too promising. So I ignored dentistry and decided on medicine. I had no idea of what the course entailed and only the vaguest ideas of what the career prospects were. To be honest, I had always had some interest in medicine in a superficial way so the decision was relatively easy in the end.

Aberdeen seemed a sensible choice for a university as it was at the terminus of the steamer and air service and as far as I knew one university was the same as another. So I applied and was accepted. I may say that I would not have been accepted today where a higher academic standard for medicine is demanded. I am not entirely sure that this is a good thing as it excludes good down to earth material and we can't all be research fellows or professors. The common sense approach to patients so necessary in general practice can only follow if the practitioner has had to overcome some of the struggles in life himself. Admittedly, some parts of medicine have become quite sophisticated and highly scientific, but it still does not help with an acute abdomen in the middle of the night, miles from laboratories or ancillary diagnostic facilities.

Having been accepted, the air force turned out to have a human face and I was allowed to clear the service two weeks early. Mind you, I was feeling quite well off now as in my last six months I was earning a bit over £3 a week. This was because the term of national service had originally been eighteen months but had been increased to two years and, I suppose as a sop for those who had unexpectedly found they had to do a further six months, the pay in the last half year was increased to match regular rates. These rates were much better than the national service rates.

So I was demobbed at Kinloss. This process took about a day and consisted of a medical examination then signatures from all over the place to say you did not hold any of their property. All the webbing, packs, etc., were handed in but the uniform was retained for future training. This would probably be a fortnight once a year. Fortunately it appeared too complicated and, probably, expensive and I was never called to do it. Like thousands of others my uniform hung in the wardrobe for years until I doubt if it would have fitted and I threw it out.

I left Kinloss on a Monday morning, took the train to Aberdeen, caught the *St Clair* to Shetland that night, spent Tuesday getting a few civilian clothes and embarked on the boat again at 6pm, arriving in Aberdeen on Wednesday morning. Fortunately I had my aunt Maggie there and had digs for the first few weeks until I got settled down.

Chapter 5

Another six

I WAS two days late. The university term started on the Monday and they had had an introductory few days the week before. I missed all that and would have been completely disorientated if it had not been for the enrolment of another Shetlander in the first year of medicine. This was Maureen Cluness, whom I did not know very well as she was now two years junior to me at school. She told me what books to get and gave me the timetable for Thursday, the following day. It started at nine with practical physics, studying optics. This was at Marischal College. The zoology department was also at Marischal but chemistry was in a new building in Old Aberdeen near Kings College, and botany in yet another building there. This meant a lot of transfers between classes either walking about half to three-quarters of a mile or waiting for a bus. I was pleased the first day at the chemistry building to discover the caretaker there was policeman Peter Walterson from Shetland; his son, Lowrie, followed on behind me in medicine the following year.

I found the physics laboratory and discovered everybody had teamed up in pairs and were busy setting up some experiments with lenses, light, mirrors, etc. I felt a bit lost but then, like a lifebelt thrown to me in the water, I heard an argument between a pair close by and the Orkney accent was quite recognisable. "Do you two come from Orkney?" I asked.

"Yes, from Stronsay."

"I am from Shetland, and seem to be the odd one out, do you mind if I join you?"

"Not at all," was the answer.

There started a friendship which exists to this day. The two were twins, Ronnie and Billy, sons of the doctor in Stronsay, who had the medically unfortunate name of Pyle. They never really accepted being addressed as 'the haemorrhoids' and who could blame them. Ronnie was the more dominant of the two, Billy the more easily likeable. They were both great characters and afforded endless amusement to myself and even more so the fourth musketeer, Martin Lees from Aberdeen, who joined us a bit later, but who knew Ronnie and Billy as they had all been at Aberdeen Grammar School together.

Billy's and Ronnie's mother had died when they were quite young so they had been sent to boarding school at the Aberdeen Grammar, only going home to Orkney for holidays. This, of course, accounted for the 'old man' personalities of these two 18-year-olds. They wore waistcoats and fob watches with chains, something I had seen my grandfather wear, but nobody since. They were very independent young men and although they were in digs together never travelled together; one would appear before the appointed time, usually Billy, and then a few minutes later the second could be seen approaching the rendezvous. Their personalities were quite different and they argued interminably. I met their father very briefly in Kirkwall once and I could see an older model of Ronnie. I presume Billy took more of his mother's genes, but of course I could only guess this.

Ronnie, Billy, Martin and I sat together at lectures, went together for coffee and went out together on Saturday nights, and that was to be the pattern for the next six years. Later in the clinical years at Foresterhill and other hospitals we were divided up onto 'clinics' of eight. This was alphabetic and thus Pyle,

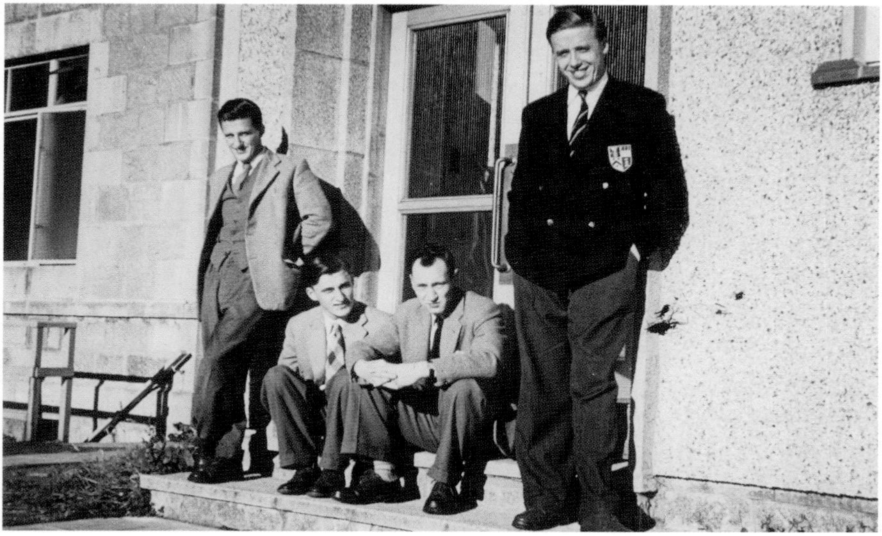

The four musketeers at Maternity Hospital, Aberdeen, whilst doing our practical obstetrics, from left: Ronnie Pyle, Billy Pyle, the author, Martin Lees.

Ritchie, Roe, Robertson, etc. came to be together in the wards; Martin being 'Lees' fell among the J to O lot so attended different wards from the two Pyles and me. Perhaps this was a blessing in disguise as Martin had the most explosive sense of humour I ever came across.

Martin Lees just could not contain himself in a funny situation. He would become quite red in the face, splutter a bit, rapidly produce a handkerchief and explode behind it, though it was poor camouflage. It was difficult in his company not to have the giggles as well and, of course, often the circumstances were not suitable. Martin enjoyed the quaint antics of the Pyles tremendously and often I have seen him double up with laughter to such an extent he ended up on the floor convulsed, and with the tears streaming down his face.

Most of the physics, particularly the radiological part of it, was new to me; the chemistry became new when we got onto organic chemistry; the botany was all new and some of the zoology. There were class examinations each term, all leading up to the degree examinations at the end of the third term. All four subjects had to be passed to go on to second year.

I had been advised by Albert Thomason, who had been a few years ahead of me at school and who was doing medicine at Edinburgh, to use a study schedule of six nights work and one off. This I proceeded to do and did so for six years, with a very occasional night off for the pictures when all four of us agreed. If one said no, he had to work, it meant we all worked. There was so much studying to be done we were afraid to lose even one evening but there seemed safety in numbers. So it was lectures and practicals all day then back to the digs, tea, and by six o'clock down to the books until about eleven o'clock. I found that after 10 o'clock I read the same line two or three times and if I honestly stopped and asked myself what I had read, I could not remember. Consequently I never worked after 11pm.

One of the class at that time was a male nurse from Glasgow. He had struggled hard to get his highers and was much older than the rest of us. He had another tremendous barrier for a student in that he was deaf and wore a hearing aid. I presume that students, even medical students, acted like members of parliament do today, and erupted in noise whenever anything displeased them. It appeared to be traditional to disrupt. Looking back I think it was rather childish. Poor Davy had to rapidly turn down the volume of his hearing aid when these noisy episodes occurred. He sat at the front of the lecture theatre to get the best reception he could and when these uproars occurred he would turn down his hearing aid and then turn round and glower at the rest of us. Poor Davy failed his botany at the end of the first year and I spent an increasingly alcoholic afternoon with him in the Kirkgate Bar after the results came out. He repeated over and over again, "Jesus Christ, just to think that two pieces of chickweed and a bloody docken could stop you from being a doctor." In true Glasgow fashion he had hit the nail on the head. Unfortunately that was the end of Davy. I expect he went back to nursing.

There were various others, some of them characters of a different type, who brought some fun to what was really a pretty serious business but who also disappeared at the end of the first year. One of these was, I think, a little insane. He climbed the Mitchell Tower at Marischal College to hang a banner for some rectorial election and left a 'po' tied to the top of the tower. He also climbed out over the wires across the Rubislaw quarry. The wires were greasy and the drop many hundreds of feet to the quarry floor. Perhaps it was just as well that he was another of those who 'disappeared'.

The summer vacation was quite long and I think we needed it to recharge the batteries. I got a job through Willie Inkster, the harbour master at Lerwick. Willie was a great Unst man and if you came from Unst or had Unst connections then you were in favour. So for many years I worked during my holidays to Lerwick Harbour Trust, and what a super crowd of men I worked with. I enjoyed it so much. It was the fresh air life and though it was, like most jobs, full of routine, there was lots of fun in among it. This was due to the boss and the splendid crew which worked for him. Lang Charlie Edwardson was the waterman, who had a cart with hoses for watering the boats. The skipper of the *Budding Rose*, the pilot boat, was Leonard Scollay. I eventually ended up as crewman to Leonard on the *Budding Rose* and what a splendid fellow he was. It was a great pleasure to be with him. He had a great sense of humour and was always considerate and kind. The pilot was Willie Smith at that time and many an hour we spent rolling about off the Bressay Light, waiting for a ship needing the pilot.

If we had to wait for a ship then we put down a hand-line. There is nothing better than a bit of sea fishing and to be able to fish from a substantial boat for a change, as well as getting paid while doing it, made that part of the job pleasurable indeed.

Very often when coming ashore late at night we were met by Willie Inkster as we tied the boat up. "Come up to the house and have a dram before you go home." A dram was always accompanied by tea or coffee and something to eat. Willie was very kind and looked after his men well. In return they had a great deal of respect for him.

One day we were sorting out some heavy, greasy wire on Victoria Pier when Willie appeared with some very important visitors whom he was showing round. Willie said, "I must introduce you to one of our men, Dr Robertson." I was obliged to shake hands with these people without trying to correct the advancement from a mere medical student which Willie had given me. I have no idea what they made of it.

First job every morning at 7am was sweeping and cleaning Alexandra Building corridors and stairs. At 9am we had time off for breakfast and how I enjoyed it. Thereafter it might be the pilot boat or usually some more mundane task like painting corrugated iron buildings with grey paint. Cleaning the marine growth off the Loofa Baa beacon and painting it was never a popular task. It was quite hard work trying to get rid of tang and growth with a hoe. At least there was some variety and it was physical, in the open air, just what I needed and wanted. I was always grateful to Willie for giving me these summer jobs.

Second year medicine was a big one with the subjects continued for two terms into the third year before the second MB examination. There were two side subjects as well as the main three in anatomy, physiology and biochemistry. I never really understood these side subjects and the class examination in statistics proved it. The examination was an hour-long paper. After a quarter of an hour I had answered what I could and there seemed no point in sitting looking into thin air so I handed in my paper and walked out to great applause from the class. All my friends had assured me they did not understand the subject either so I thought I had given them the lead. I sat for the remaining three quarters of the hour on the step outside the examination hall but nobody appeared. I thought I had cooked my goose and when the lecturer came in some days later he announced that some people had done a good paper but some had not. In fact one student had managed to get one per cent. I turned to my pals and with some pride said, "That's me!"

However, I had got 15 per cent and Billy Pyle, who had spent the whole hour, got 12 per cent. I never did find out who the brilliant student was who got the booby prize for one per cent. Genetics was also badly taught and proved to be a side subject with poor marks in the class examination for a lot of us.

Biochemistry, which dealt with the chemical processes in the body, appeared extremely difficult and complex to begin with, whereas physiology (how the body works) looked quite straightforward. However, as time went on biochemistry began to come together quite nicely, whereas physiology became the most difficult subject in the entire medical course. I well remember one of the questions in the degree examination in biochemistry – 'Discuss the nutritive value of a meal of fish and chips'. I wrote pages at the time but would have some difficulty in doing so now.

The practical physiology was interesting when we did the experiments. Things like stimulating muscular contraction in frogs' legs by means of a small electrical impulse on a nerve, or bathing a mammalian heart in an infusion to which various things were added and the resultant variation recorded, are two of the many I can still remember. The teaching was not very good and we depended on a really good text book. The one I used was by Sampson Wright and it had many small but interesting paragraphs which were much more interesting than the main bulk of the book. One such paragraph recorded a case of a man in America who went a whole year without a bowel movement. It did not say how this concrete example was remedied but he did survive. We all found this item quite fascinating and none of us ever worried about constipation thereafter.

During our time in biochemistry we had to do a dietary survey on ourselves for seven days. This meant weighing and noting everything we ate and drank for a week. We all carried notebooks and nutritional tables and noted down every cup of coffee and every biscuit as well as the main meals. This all had to be analysed in large columns of figures and an analytic study of the results presented. It was an awful lot of work but was allowed 20 per cent of the degree examination mark, so was absolutely vital.

I came in one morning proudly stating I had completed my dietary survey the previous evening. I had 4,000 calories/day. Nobody else got much over 3,000 and I began to worry about the accuracy of my results. When I came to analyse them again I found that porridge every morning with layers of sugar and milk, and three spoons of sugar in every cup of tea (of which there were many during the day) pushed this excessive calorific intake to this high level. I got a good mark for my survey.

The professor of biochemistry at that time was Professor Kermack. He had been blinded in a laboratory accident many years before. No doubt he was a brilliant man, but an awful lecturer. It did not help that he used slides projected on a screen and pointed quite accurately with a pointer to the various stages of biochemical changes. One day I was astounded to see Professor Kermack drive a car out of the quadrangle and through the rather narrow gate at Marischal College into Broad Street. All was revealed next day when a visiting professor from USA was introduced. He had a left-hand-drive car.

Anatomy was the main subject. We had a lecture every morning in anatomy from 9am to 10am. Thereafter we were supposed to go directly to 'the drain'. The drain was the anatomical dissection room where six students shared a corpse. These corpses were a bit shrivelled and smelt very, very strongly of formaldehyde in which they had been preserved for a long time. Mainly homeless down and outs I think. At the end of the dissection there was a burial service in the department which we all attended and the bits and pieces were given a Christian burial. Formaldehyde is a pungent fluid which catches and stings the mucous membranes of your nose and throat. After a few days it became less of a problem and eventually we only noticed it in the morning when we went in to start the day's dissection. It took all the first term just to do head and neck as every nerve, artery, vein, muscle, ligament, tendon and lymph node had to be carefully displayed. It meant hours and hours of careful picking, scraping and cutting and the morning's work for six would be hardly noticeable from the previous day's exploration.

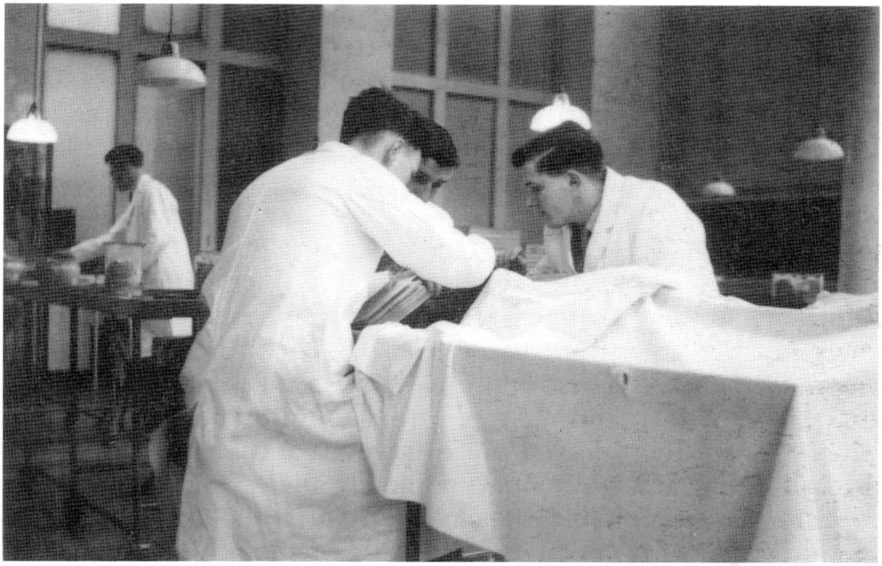

Dissecting the body in the anatomy department, from left: the author, Billy Pyle, Ronnie Pyle.

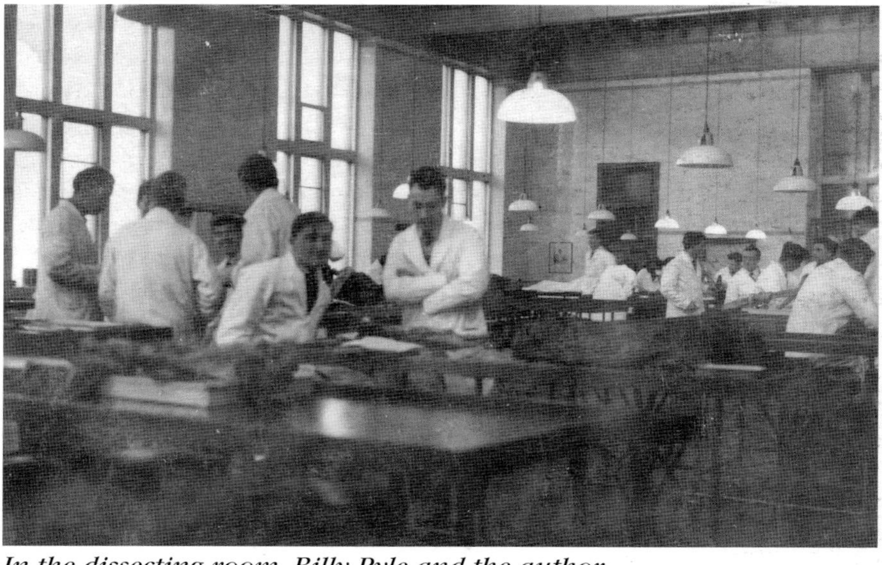

In the dissecting room, Billy Pyle and the author.

At the end of the first three weeks in anatomy, we received a considerable shock with the first 'spotter examination'. This took place in the dissection room, a large room in which a huge circle of tables was set out. Each student was given a number and told to go to the table of that number. If your number was 29 you started at table 29, and eventually ended up answering question 28. A bell rang and one minute was allowed to read the questions at the table, decide what the lump of grey tissue was and where it came from, then identify the small numbered flags, usually about three of them. Alternatively you might be asked to list three flags demonstrating some structures from half a dozen stuck into the specimen. It seemed impossible to orientate the specimen, read the question and answer in the minute allowed. The bell rang and you then moved on to table 30 and so on. Of course, when the first few were not completely answered, the panic set in and on further tables it was even worse. In this circle five lecturers sat with specimens in front of them and they asked direct questions. We all carried long dissection forceps and the appropriate vein, nerve, muscle or whatever had to be picked up with the forceps. This was also a shambles, making things worse still. I got 33 per cent, nothing like a pass but most of us were in the same boat. This looked like the end of the line for many, including myself.

There was much discussion and a great deal of anxiety. A completely different approach was obviously required. From then on we looked at each body in the drain as each was slightly different. We formed twos and fired questions at each other over the appropriate dissection area. Show me this, show me that, what structure is this, what lies behind it, etc., etc. Anatomy illustrations always showed arteries in red, veins in blue, lymphatics in green, nervous tissue in white, etc., but these specimens we worked with were uniformly grey. The next spotter was difficult, but so much easier after the new approach and from then on, no more failures.

Anatomy was logical and just required a lot of memory work. It never really posed a problem to me after the initial start. We spent from 10am to 1pm every day for five terms doing dissection.

The professor of anatomy was an old, crotchety bachelor by the name of Lockhart. We rarely saw him except for the lectures he gave between 9 and 10am.

Having been two years in the RAF, I needed my NAAFI break after the 9-10am lecture and, like most of us, ran across to the Students' Union for a coffee and a bun before going to the drain. One day on returning we were met by the professor in the doorway. "Well, well, well, and where have you young people been?"

"At the Union for a cup of coffee, sir," I replied. I probably would have said nothing but I could see that this was the crunch, and I could not function from 8am until 1pm without some coffee and a bun, so I was going to fight to get it.

"Do you mean to say that you are drinking coffee when you should be working? What would your parents think of that?"

"My parents would encourage me to have something to eat, sir" I found myself replying.

The professor turned on his heel and went off scratching his head and muttering to himself. To give him his due, he never asked again and the coffee-break continued all the time we did anatomy.

Many years later, after graduation, I was in Aberdeen and went to the anatomy department to see one of my year, George Robertson, who was then demonstrator in the department. George said, "You will have to say hello to the Professor. He always likes to see any former student. He has a photograph and all your details which he looks up before he sees you."

I went in to see Professor Lockhart and, of course, he was very nice. Whether it said 'Coffee Rebel' on my file, I don't know.

"In the first war I was a doctor on a destroyer and many a time I was in Stornoway," he said. All I could do was to appear interested and asked him what he thought of it. I can't remember the reply, which was irrelevant anyway.

How many people, even the top academics like him, think that Shetland is somewhere in the Hebrides? Eventually you get to the stage where you don't even correct them.

There were three lecturers including the professor in the department and three or four demonstrators. The latter were doctors studying anatomy before proceeding to the FRCS examination, i.e. a higher surgical qualification. They naturally did not take it so seriously so that the oral part of the spotter examination was more relaxed with them.

Another side subject at this time under the anatomy department was embryology. This was really the anatomy of the foetus. In the class examination there was a question – 'Describe a human afterbirth'. One Nigerian student, who went by the magnificent name of Percy Palgrave Shaftsbury Nylander, wrote pages on: 'It has a face with two eyes, a nose, a mouth and two ears, two legs and two arms ... ' He kept on repeating, "But how can that be? How can that be?" when he got zero marks for his answer. I don't know if he ever did understand why, even after having the difference between afterbirth and after birth, as one and two words, explained to him .

The oral degree examinations in anatomy were divided into red and blue. If you got over 60 per cent in the written papers and your 'spotter' results were satisfactory, you were allocated a blue oral examination. This meant you had already passed and I was very relieved to find I had a blue. The oral was just a formality. One demonstrator asked me to show him a nose! It was intensive interrogation for the poor reds however. One student was asked a deep anatomical question by the professor and obviously did not know. He then asked him a simpler question on some muscle attachment parts on a bone. Still no reasonable answers. "Right then, can you show me the skin of the back?" He did, but was never seen again.

It was a great relief to me to receive a red card after the second MB examination. Let me explain the significance of a red card. When the examination results were ready, the word passed round like wild-fire among the waiting candidates and they rushed across to Marischal College to queue up at the porter's box. You gave your name and he sorted through the pile of cards then presented it to you face down. There is no easy way to get examination results, but this was like poker. On turning the card over, the print on it was all red, all black, or a mixture of both. The candidate has satisfied the examiners in anatomy, physiology and biochemistry and has passed each subject: all in red. A failure in one or more was printed in black. As the reader can see, a rapid glance at the colour immediately told your fortune. There was an opportunity to re-sit the examinations later in the summer but failure of the re-sit meant the end or, if lucky, a chance to repeat the year. Re-sits allowed no summer work so were an economic disaster as well as having to spend the summer vacation studying. To repeat a year was even worse. It meant seven years instead of six before graduation, friends moved on and the repeat had to start making contacts all over again. And what was really critical was the possibility of no grant from the local education authority. Your future probably then depended on the willingness and ability of parents to pay, and few could.

Throughout my six years at Aberdeen, there was a firm insistence on attendance. A roll call was taken every morning in anatomy and when the clinical part of the course at the medical school at Foresterhill and in the various hospital wards started, it was also a daily occurrence. We were broken up into small groups for ward work and the first thing each day was a check on who was there. A few absences required a visit to the professor to explain yourself. As far as I know the medical faculty was the only one in the university to do this. On starting university, the schoolboy or girl immediately became an adult and was treated as such. It was entirely up to the individual student to attend classes and to do the required studying or not as they saw fit. It was a chasm which some found they could not cross.

Some of my fellow medical students objected to these checks on attendance, stating they were not school children and did not like being treated as such. The vast majority of us would not have missed lectures or ward rounds under any circumstance. Those who did miss the ward work in particular, rarely lasted the course. I think the philosophy at Aberdeen was: attend all ward rounds for three years and the potential doctor will be reasonably safe to be let loose on the general public, provided he passes the set examinations. We took the whole thing very seriously indeed.

The doctors in the hospital tended to be polite and pleasant teachers on the whole but some were very sarcastic and could make the student very uncomfortable. 'Clinics' consisted of eight students, divided up into alphabetical groups so, for example, P, R, S, surnames got stuck together. One of my fellow students was called Smythe and he was a pompous little man. At roll call in the ward the doctor called the roll and read out, "Smith."

"Smythe, sir, not Smith."

The tutor looked long and hard at Smythe over his glasses then, to our great enjoyment said, "Smith or Smythe, shit or shite, it's all the same to me."

However, I am getting ahead of the next stage after the second MB when the move was made from Marischal College up to Foresterhill to start the clinical years.

Chapter 6

Reality

THE clinical part of the course was now about to start and at last we felt we were to become real medical students. All the lectures were now at Foresterhill, at the medical school just across the road from the Infirmary. Practical classes in bacteriology, pathology and materia medica were also held there, so for half the day we were in the medical school and the other half in the wards. The tools of the trade now had to be acquired from Whitelaw, the surgical outfitter at Woolmanhill. Here we purchased stethoscope, tendon hammer, tape measure, oroscope, ophthalmoscope, pencil torch, and a combined instrument of brush on one end and sharp point on the other. This required some sort of case to carry it all as well as lecture notebooks. This case went everywhere and had to stand up to three years hard wear.

There were four main sites where we saw patients: Foresterhill, the main hospital and medical school; Woodend Hospital about a mile further west of Foresterhill; Woolmanhill in the centre of the city which had various outpatient clinics and the accident and emergency centre; and the City Hospital right down at the beach. Moving from one centre to the other required some time and at least one bus journey. Dr Needham, one of the medical consultants at Woodend, asked the question the first day we were there, "What is the most important piece of equipment which a medical student should possess?" None of the answers we gave were right and eventually he said, "An old pushbike."

This was correct in a way, but was really a sarcastic remark on our arrival time at Woodend for ward work. Always there was a lecture at Foresterhill from 9am to 10am. He expected us to be at Woodend by 10.15am. This was not possible as the two alternatives were to walk the mile or so between, or walk a quarter of a mile to catch a bus which was quite infrequent at that time of day. We always walked and always stopped at the cafe at Woodend for a coffee on the way.

Bacteriology and pathology were well taught, although rather dull subjects with many hours spent peering down microscopes in the hope that at the end of a year the appropriate few cells or bacteria would be recognisable when the third MB examination took place. Attendance at post mortems was part of the pathology course and, though unpleasantly smelly, proved to be quite fascinating. Materia medica, or therapeutics, was an important part of the course but the department was a bit old fashioned. For example, we spent three lectures on alcohol and one or two on antibiotics. Practical consisted of making an infusion of quassia and totally irrelevant procedures of that kind, soon to be forgotten and never seen or heard of since.

The all important subjects of medicine and surgery now constituted the first lecture each morning and would continue until the end of the sixth year, in conjunction with the subjects being studied that year (in the case of third year and fourth, the subjects just mentioned).

The lectures on medicine were very well delivered on the whole, particularly when the Professor of Medicine, Professor Fullerton, gave the lecture. He was clear and methodical and fortunately he gave most of the morning lectures. The surgical lectures tended to be more entertaining but not so easily digested, the showman not always being the best teacher.

We were expected from now on to come back to the hospital in the evenings to stand around and observe, either in casualty or in operating theatres watching operations. This was voluntary and we did attend from time to time but could not really afford the time away from the books in the evening. A little bit of practical experience was fine but at the end of the day it was the examinations which counted. Many an evening was spent hanging round and sometimes seeing or being told very little. It depended on how busy the receiving doctors were and how inclined they were to teach.

Another degree examination in these three subjects to pass, then on to the next stage: public health, very dry and not very interesting; psychology, which might have been interesting but was taught, it seemed to us, in a foreign language, so unfortunately we made little sense of it. (It was not until years later, doing a refresher course at Oxford, that I began to understand it. Of course, it is more relevant when older and having dealt with people for some time, but the lectures at Oxford were superb); forensic medicine was a new and fascinating subject and the lecturer, who was police surgeon at Aberdeen, excellent. Just before the degree examination at the end of the year he did something which never happened to us before or again. He gave us a broad hint that it might be advisable to make sure we knew all about gunshot wounds. Right enough, one of the questions in the paper was on just that.

The side subjects were now started as well: ear, nose and throat; skin; venereal disease; eyes; psychiatry; orthopaedics; social medicine; etc. At the same time, surgery and medicine continued in the wards. Later on we were introduced to gynaecology and obstetrics.

Many of the lecturers from the hospital were characters, the surgeons being a bit more flamboyant than the physicians. As I have said, there were eight students to each clinic. Thus the same eight were attached to a ward and on arrival we were delegated cases. We then had an hour to take a full history from the patient and examine them, before the registrar or consultant appeared and cast the dice. You always hoped it would not be your patient which turned up, but it really was decided on which clinical material was most instructive for the student.

The more difficult and sarcastic consultants could make quite a fool of the student in front of his seven colleagues, and the patient. "All right, Mr P., you think this patient is suffering from such and such. What are you going to give him to treat the condition?"

Mr P. considered for a while then said, "Tincture of X."

"How much, and how often?" he was asked.

Again a long pause then, "One minim twice a day, sir."

There was a small explosion from the consultant who threw the case notes down on the bed. "Christ boy, you might as well pee in the ocean and expect the tide to rise!"

Some of the answers in the therapeutics paper were highly amusing. One comes to mind even to this day. The question was: "Write prescriptions for the following". One of the list was pyelitis, i.e. inflammation of the kidney. The student obviously did not know what pyelitis was as he wrote: "Tincture of iodine – paint the affected part three times a day."

Another on the list was oxyuriasis. At the time I did not know what this was, only after the examination discovering it was a type of worm infection. I remember thinking, 'Oxyuriasis? Must have something to do with urine, so oxy must be air in the urine'. It would have been just as amusing to the examiner who told us about the pyelitis to have read out my remedy for 'gassy urine'.

Having been delegated a young girl from Orkney one day at Woodend I drew the short straw with one of the more sarcastic consultants. I went through her case history and had started to read out the results of my examination. The poor girl was sitting up on the bed stripped to the waist. "Respiratory system: the trachea is central, the chest moves well on inspiration ..."

He interrupted me at this point asking, "Show me which part of the chest you like to see moving."

I did not know what the correct answer was so put a finger just above each breast.

"You must have a dirty mind, boy."

The rest of the clinic were greatly amused, I was not and still don't know what the correct answer was.

One surgeon who was well known for his sarcasm listened to one of our group go through his case history and then what he had found on examination, interrupting from time to time and making the going tough for this particular student. Eventually he asked, "So, what's your diagnosis?"

The student produced one of the little known conditions normally printed in small print at the foot of a page in the textbook.

"Come here and look out this window." We were in a ward on the second floor at Foresterhill. "Do you see any birds?"

"Yes, sir, there is a seagull."

"Clever boy, so it is. You are much more likely to see one out of these windows than a flamingo." It was a good point and well worth remembering in practice.

No doubt when a lecturer found a good line he repeated it to each new class. It was a great help, if the subject was rather dull, if the lecturer interspersed his talk with some wit. Probably it was the wit we remembered rather than the serious content. Apart from the odd bit of humour, lectures at this stage were heard in silence. All the background noise of early years was now considered puerile, as indeed it was.

Almost every student wrote furiously as the lecture was delivered. It depended on the speed of delivery, but most of these notes took a fair bit of reading afterwards. To sit and scribble at speed for six years meant an almost indecipherable scrawl and in my opinion contributed to the well known bad writing of doctors.

One consultant started his 9am lecture off one day with: "Many famous people died young; Mozart died young. So did Napoleon and Alexander the Great, and I am not feeling well myself." He was well known to us for his wit and sense of humour, but at the same time was a bit pompous and vain and so the joke was really a bit two edged.

Venereology was in a small department at outpatients at Woolmanhill, the old Aberdeen infirmary, near HM Theatre and the Cowdray Hall. There was one consultant there and I think he may have had a registrar, but I can only remember him. He was Dr Bowie, who originated from Shetland. Clinics in his department were very relaxed affairs for us students, though I doubt if they were for the poor patient. He always threw down a packet of cigarettes and a lighter and told us to help ourselves. He, of course, puffed away as well, before the patient came in. Changed days.

Dr Bowie's lectures were once a week, just after lunch at Foresterhill Medical School. He always appeared in a taxi in his white coat and he introduced his subject and his first lecture as follows: "Good afternoon, ladies and gentlemen. So you want to learn something about the pox, do you?"

A great cheer and a loud "Yes" answered that.

"The first thing that you must learn is never trust anybody. Why, only yesterday I had a minister come to see me and he asked, 'Is it possible, doctor, to get VD off a public lavatory seat?' "

"Yes, it is," I replied, "but it is a filthy place to take a young lady."

The skin department was another relaxed place and the consultant was a very nice man who no doubt knew his subject well, but unfortunately he was not a great teacher. Every skin lesson was "erythematous dermatitis with mild papular and vesicular manifestations" or so it seemed to us at the time. It was only with the aid of a good dermatology text book and an excellent atlas of skin lesions that I managed to deal with dermatological problems in general practice. Gradually you got a feel for the subject and became much better in diagnosis and treatment. Like everything else, experience seemed to be the secret and luckily skin problems rarely were acute emergencies.

Ophthalmology was a subject that did not seem to be well taught. Part of the problem was mastering the ophthalmoscope. This is a hand-held instrument with an arrangement of lenses and mirrors with a light source. While looking through one of the

a very good teacher he liked having students around. He sometimes asked me a question and one day, assisting at a nephrectomy (removal of a kidney), but before we had reached the renal pelvis, he asked me to tell him the relationship of the various structures at the renal pelvis. I got it wrong, much to my embarrassment, with all the theatre staff and the GP anaesthetist listening. "Always remember," Charles said, "Virgins Are Useless." I thought he was getting too much of the ether which circulated in quantity in theatre in those days. He then proceeded to explain, "Vein, Artery, Ureter, from anterior to posterior." I never forgot that anatomical relationship.

I mentioned Robbie Robertson the diver earlier. He was in the Old Gilbert Bain as a patient at that time. After a ward round one day with Charles Anderson, sitting in his room having coffee, he asked me if I knew Robbie, and if he was a relation. I said yes, he was a grand uncle of mine and I knew him quite well. "He is in hospital with a bad back and do you know what he told me when I asked him if he had ever injured his back? 'Oh yes,' Robbie had immediately answered, 'I hurt it out in the China Sea many years ago. We were in a three-masted ship and got caught in a typhoon. We were dismasted so the skipper told me to take a hundred coolies, go ashore, and cut down appropriate trees for new masts. Well, we were on the way back to the ship carrying this huge tree when the mate blew the whistle for dinner and they all ran off leaving me carrying the tree, and I have had a bad back ever since.' "

Fortunately Charles Anderson enjoyed the story, which Robbie had told him in all seriousness.

Assisting Charles operating was easier after a time. He was slow spoken with an Aberdeenshire accent and he operated slowly, deliberately and carefully, in the same way as he spoke. After he left Shetland to go to Arbroath, I assisted Ronnie Cumming, the new consultant surgeon, for a short period. Ronnie spoke very quickly, out of the side of his mouth with his Highland accent, and his operating was just as rapid as his speech. Not only did he speak quickly, but it was not always easy to understand what he said, especially with a mask on and his head bent over the patient's abdomen, a few inches below mine.

The few staff in the hospital in those days always seemed to cope without any great signs of stress. Matron was Jean Innes, theatre sister was initially Sister Christie, I think from Burra Isle - I remember her as tall and rather severe. She was later replaced by Jess Andrews who was friendly, helpful and efficient but with a good sense of humour, making life in theatre so much more pleasant, especially for a mere medical student.

It was about this time that I met my future wife. I was hauling up the yoal, which gave me so much fun in the summer holidays, at Craigie Stane at the South End. Maureen was at that time a midwife in the 'Annexe' at the foot of Lover's Loan. This had been a 'wrenery' during the war and consisted of a row of parallel Nissan huts connected together by concrete steps in a corridor. Steps were required because the huts were stepped up the hill behind Midgarth. The midwives' accommodation was in huts on the other side of the Loan. Maureen stopped and watched my boat hauling efforts then offered to help. I promptly declined this female offer.

Later we met again and she gave me some practical experience in the Annexe in bathing babies, so that this did not terrify me the way it did Ronnie Pyle at a later date.

Maureen invited me to the Annexe Christmas party that year and I felt a bit shy when I appeared at it. I always remember that it was not those whom I knew who put me at my ease, but Neil Cadenhead who came across and welcomed me in. That kindness I never forgot.

I enjoyed gynaecology, but even more so obstetrics. In the later years of the medical course the great decision has to be made between a career in hospital or in general practice. I had leaned towards the latter and it was only when I did obstetrics that I had some doubts as to which I should pursue. The options were still open at that stage, but it would have to be one or the other.

We were always being advised, quite correctly, by the university students' health service to do some sport. I found that there was little time to spare for it and anyway I was not very good at it. My digs were in Hilton Avenue and my landlady was a German woman whom we called 'Ma Anderson'. Shortly after I moved into these digs, Drew Tulloch joined me and, being a good friend, fairly enlivened what was a pretty routine, dull existence of work with more work. It was difficult to get to Foresterhill from Hilton Avenue unless by bus into the town then transfer to another and come out again, so I decided to walk and this I did every morning and evening for the rest of my university days. I enjoyed it, especially in the morning, and it took about half an hour so it was a reasonable distance.

Drew and I had some good fun in among the rest with Ma Anderson. She was a well meaning lady, who spoke with a strong German accent. Her son lived upstairs in the house with his wife Katy, who came from Skye. She had a good sense of humour and it was always like a breath of fresh air to go upstairs and chat with Katy.

Ma Anderson never really understood students and having little sense of humour and no sense of smell was always open to practical jokes. She was always intensely curious if we did anything different from the routine. I had arranged to buy a half skeleton from another student so this meant an evening excursion to collect it. Ma was eaten up with curiosity as to why and where I was going after tea. She made it so obvious that she played directly into our hands.

"I am going to the anatomy department to collect a bit of a corpse to do some work on at home," I told her when her ceaseless enquiries could not be put off any longer.

Drew, of course, knew the truth and when I came back with a cardboard box with the half skeleton, he immediately turned up his nose and said, "What a smell."

"Where are you going to keep it?" I was asked.

"Oh, underneath my bed, in my suitcase."

I had to put the imaginary body parts in there as it could lock and it would prevent Ma from finding out when she searched our room next day, as we knew she would. She was not at all subtle and tended to move things or leave drawers disturbed. Katy upstairs was in on the joke and would make remarks with a turned up nose about the strange smell downstairs. We kept this up for a few days until Ma's many daughters all knew about it and the news began to spread. I thought it might even get back to the university authorities and decided the 'body' would have to go back. Next morning, some twigs out of the garden wrapped in a bit of brown paper with were carried very obviously when I went out. Naturally, she could not refrain from asking what the parcel was and I told her.

This had worked so well Drew and I went to the Joke Factory in George Street and purchased some stink bombs. The bathroom was between our bedroom, where we studied at night, and the kitchen, where Ma spent her evenings. We waited until she went to the bathroom. We went in immediately after and set off a stink bomb. The next part of the fun was to make a lot of noise and fuss outside the bathroom and at the foot of the stairs. Katy then appeared, as did Ma, and it ended up with Ma marching round the bathroom with rolls of lighted newspaper to dispel the smell she could not detect.

At one stage she set two mousetraps in the kitchen before she went to bed. Drew hit on the idea of removing the cheese but then re-setting the traps as we were always up later than Ma. She was amazed how clever these mice were and told everybody who came in about them.

Each evening we had our tea in the kitchen with our landlady. There was a couch alongside the table. When about to eat, Ma would pop out her false teeth and put them on the couch. I honestly think she thought she was being very discreet and that we weren't aware. One night I kicked Drew under the table and nodded my head towards the couch. Ma's cat was up licking her teeth on the couch. Ma was busy speaking and did not notice. She wondered why we were not going through to our bedroom to work immediately after tea as usual. In fact, she asked a couple of times, "Are you boys not going to study tonight?" We were delaying until the now cleaned dentures were restored to their rightful place.

The food in our digs was not very exciting. Yellow fish appeared at least twice a week with the result I swore I would never eat it again. I did eventually, many years later, but it never became an item of choice on my menu.

Drew graduated BSc Engineering after three years, and I was left on my own again.

When the final examinations started then applications for the first house job in hospital had to be considered. The top jobs were the wards of professors and the most eminent consultants in the teaching hospital. These jobs went to the medal winners in the class or those with distinction. This was the path which those who aspired to academic distinction would follow. Lesser graduates took or applied for the other jobs, some of which were much sought after and others not. We lesser mortals felt that the top jobs offered less responsibility, the houseman being the office boy, expected to make the tea. I doubt if that was a correct assumption, but it was believed at that time. I got a job in Ear, Nose and Throat, provided of course I could display the degree of MB ChB when the time came.

The finals took place over two weeks. Firstly the written examinations, in medicine, surgery, gynaecology and obstetrics. Then the practical examinations; each student was given cases to check and examine in the wards and was grilled on them by the examiner. Finally, and worst of all, the oral examinations. By the time the final oral examinations took place we had had experience of them in every degree subject throughout the six years, but the terror did not diminish. The technique, however, improved. Waiting to be called needed a full pack of cigarettes and a convenient toilet. Name called, open door, see three professors or equivalent seated opposite the door at a table, advance, say good morning or equivalent, be invited to sit down opposite, cross your fingers and appear alert, calm and, if possible, intelligent. A nice examiner would smile and ask the first question. If he was very kind, he asked a fairly straightforward question. Having answered this first question, some of the twisting came out of the gut and the rest of this period of torture might not be too bad.

I decided early to adopt an honest approach. The examiners knew the correct answers and any amount of bluffing was transparent to them. If I did not know I said so. This ended the agony and perhaps the next question would be easily answered, even though some points had been lost with the first. It always seemed to pay off for me.

In my oral in medicine, the visiting examiner came from Edinburgh. He asked a trick question, the pitfall of which I was aware, so I answered correctly. He however persisted in trying to get me to change my mind. I always considered this to be unfair. There was no smile from this gentleman, and little did I realise I would meet up with him again.

What a relief and sense of achievement to get the red card after the finals. An all night party developed but strangely did not seem to be a really joyous one. Perhaps the strain had been more than we thought, and it was not possible to relax enough.

Provisional registration with the medical governing body, the General Medical Council, was the next necessary step. At the end of the period spent in hospital, provided the boss in each job had no objection, then full registration would be applied for.

The other mandatory requirement before any kind of work was registration with the Medical Defence Society.

Graduation was a kind of assembly line, up to a platform in the Mitchell Hall with gown and mortar board, then photographs, followed by a good lunch. I remember the lunch in the Royal Athaneum Restaurant (then considered to the best place in Aberdeen), rather than the rest of the ceremony.

Two weeks holiday followed, then starting as a houseman in the hospital at the very bottom of the medical ladder. During those pre-registration jobs a final decision would have to be made between specialisation and general practice, and the appropriate choice of job sought, particularly as regards the former.

cups and a tablecloth appeared in sister's office. We, the residents, had to put on a clean white coat, and when the great man appeared he had to be welcomed at the door. After coffee, my job was to hold his stethoscope and, when he held out his hand (he did not ask, just made the signal), I presented it to him. He listened, made a comment, and I got the instrument back again. Sister pushed a trolley with the patients' notes and the two consultants and the other houseman made up the party. It took a couple of hours to do the ward round and sometime long after lunchtime he put on his heavy coat, Homburg hat and gloves and we all stood round the car until he departed. It was very cold to stand with only a thin cotton white coat on that winter, waiting for the great man to go. He had a most annoying habit of getting into his car, starting the engine then lowering his window and discussing something with one of the consultants for five or ten minutes while we slowly froze. This man was the visiting examiner in my medical oral at Aberdeen who had tried to get me to change my mind on a correct answer; I did not warm to J.D.S. Cameron on that occasion and even less so during these 'royal' visits to Peel.

Now and again the consultants were called to do domiciliary consultations. The houseman was often asked to accompany him to do an electrocardiograph. On one of these visits in Hawick the GP asked me what I intended to do. When I said general practice he told me I must get a gimmick to be successful in practice. He wore always a rose in his buttonhole. I never got round to finding a gimmick.

After five months in the job, Dr Borthwick asked me what job I had in mind when I finished at Peel. I really wanted to do a job in obstetrics, but they were difficult to get at that time, so really did not think I would be successful, especially applying from a provincial hospital in competition with the teaching hospital candidates. Dr Borthwick said he knew Dr Richard de Soldenoff in Ayrshire and that he would have a word with him. This must have been the 'old boy network', for imagine my surprise when he told me later I had an interview with Dr de Soldenoff next

Monday at the Ayrshire Central Hospital in Irvine. He had even worked out the train times for me – Galashiels to Edinburgh, Edinburgh to Glasgow, Glasgow to Irvine – and, furthermore, I had the day off to go. I was very grateful for this opportunity. It was an illustration of the type of kindness and consideration for which Jake Borthwick was well known.

And so I arrived at Irvine and made my way to the hospital. "Dr de Soldenoff is having his lunch but will see you while he eats it," I was told, and I was duly ushered into a small side room.

Dr de Soldenoff was scooping up some soup from a soup plate and told me to sit down. He was very pleasant and asked some questions while he dumped the next course into the same soup plate and then the sweet also. I was quite fascinated and my eyes almost popped out of my head when he took a cup across to

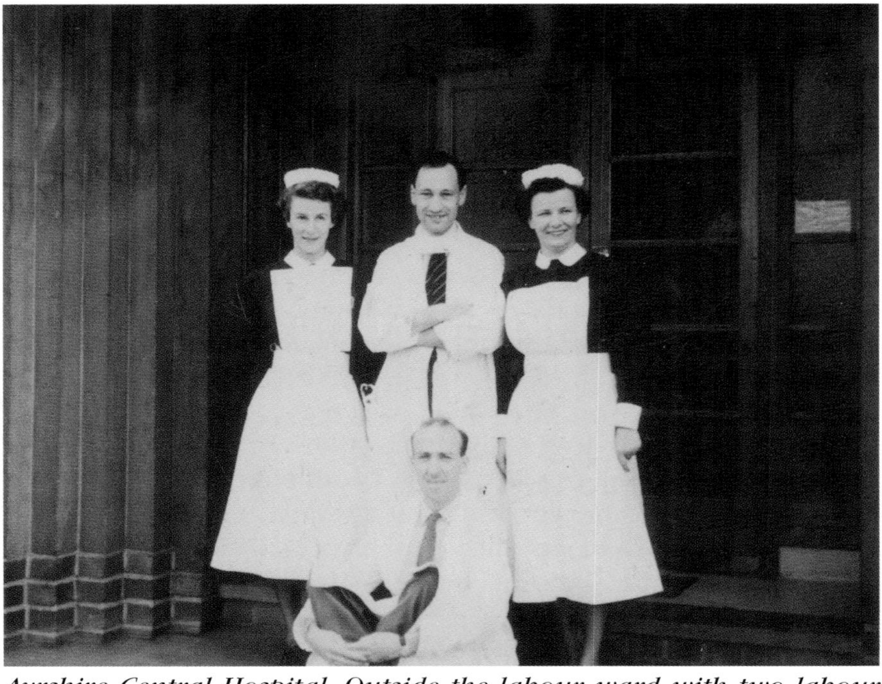

Ayrshire Central Hospital. Outside the labour ward with two labour ward sisters and, seated, Dr Stewart, one of the other residents.

the steriliser which was boiling and through a drainage tap, made his coffee.

At the end of all this he asked what time my train back was and when I told him he said, "Right, come and I will run you down to the station."

This was something new to me, a consultant running a junior house doctor to the station. Just before I got out he said, "We will look forward to seeing you in a month's time." That meant I had got the job.

When I finished at Peel, I moved directly to the west of Scotland to start the new job. It was much less formal on the Glasgow side than it had been in the Edinburgh region. There was a happy atmosphere in the hospital, partly due to the lack of formality, but mainly because both senior medical and all nursing staff were friendly, fine people to work with.

The twenty-four hours spent on 'duty one', i.e. all admissions to the hospital and labour ward responsibility, was very demanding of stamina. There was never more than half an hour to sit down apart from rushed meals so that by 4am I was like a robot. The job was extremely interesting and rewarding, as well as very instructive, until that time in the early morning. Then it was a case of dragging the sore feet to the next job where the interest was as jaded as the house officer. If I had been able to rearrange the rota I would have introduced night duty and night duty only, for a week, so a reasonable sleep and rest could recharge the batteries. As it was, after 9am there was still a day's work ahead though nothing like so intensive.

There were four housemen, four registrars, a senior registrar and two consultants at Irvine. Duty rota for the housemen was, day one: admissions and labour ward; day two: flying squad and anaesthetics; day three: antenatal and blood cross-matching; day four: postnatal and a half-day.

The idea of having to give anaesthetics was very alarming. Medical student experience of anaesthetics was minimal and then only under instruction. Here the job was explained by one of the more senior housemen. The apparatus and the various agents were crude but standard, so fortunately only short procedures needed our inexpert services.

All caesarean sections were done under a 'cocktail' of three drugs given pre-operatively and once in theatre the patient's abdomen was infiltrated with local anaesthetic working through the various abdominal strata to the peritoneum over the uterus. All housemen at Irvine were rewarded if they had done a satisfactory job by being allowed to do a caesarean section towards the end of their six months.

Our anaesthetics were given for minor procedures such as inevitable abortion, with another houseman on the other end. Artificial rupture of the membranes to start labour off became the side job for the houseman on 'duty three'. All the forceps deliveries were done under pudendal block of local anaesthetic. I did over 50 during my six months and this was to stand me in good stead. If blood was required for transfusion, one of the housemen had to cross-match it in a small laboratory before it was sent up to theatre.

One of the registrars was an Aberdeen graduate and he took a special interest in me so that I picked up a lot of extra knowledge from him. He had a house in Irvine and I spent many half-days with him and his wife who was also a medical graduate of Aberdeen. Furthermore, one of my fellow residents acquired his first car while at Irvine and, of course, we could never be off together so he gave me his car on my half-days. What between the use of the car, trips all over Ayrshire on flying squad call, and visits to outlying antenatal classes, I saw almost all of Ayrshire. It was a fine summer to add icing to the cake.

Dr de Soldenoff was a showman of the nicest kind. He had been a prisoner of the Japanese during the war and probably that was why I was shown the one plate lunch and coffee made from the steriliser. One day during a ward round with him the patients had just finished lunch and the plates were on the bed tables at the end of the beds. He suddenly stopped at one table and told the patient she had left the best part of her meal. This was the fatty bits which she had cut off. He then proceeded to stand and eat these pieces one by one until the plate was clean.

It was always pleasant to go out in his Austin Princess on flying squad calls. He wore a bowler hat, dark jacket and pinstriped trousers and always had a carnation in his button hole. This always seemed to impress the local doctor, the household, and all the neighbours who normally collected when a drama like this was unfolding. The doctor's car and the ambulance in a council estate attracted attention. All the doors in the vicinity would be open with usually two roller-haired matrons standing in each. All became quiet as Richard de Soldenoff stepped slowly out of the large black limousine, dusted himself down, rearranged his carnation, reached into the car for his bowler hat, put it on, and only then, speaking to me in a nonchalant way, went up the path to the GP anxiously waiting on the doorstep. Remember, this was an emergency situation.

I carried in the many cases and boxes which comprised the flying squad equipment and we got to work. When the patient was resuscitated sufficiently she was transferred to the waiting ambulance while we packed up and left. Only then did the entertainment for the entire street finish.

At a later stage I was sometimes sent on flying squad call by myself, accompanied only by a midwife, but this depended on the type and seriousness of the incident.

I remember one such case on a Saturday night. We were called to a very obese, relatively young woman, well on in her pregnancy, who was suffering from eclampsia. She had had two or three fits before we arrived at the council estate in Kilmarnock. The patient was in a bedroom where we proceeded to sedate her and check her blood pressure prior to transfer to the hospital. It took us a couple of hours before she was fit for the journey but meantime a riotous, drunken party went on in the other part of the house. Nobody seemed to be in the slightest way concerned about the patient, so much so that we transferred her to the ambulance without anybody even coming to the door. The patient survived to go back to whatever kind of life she had.

Most of the worst cases we admitted at Irvine came from Saltcoats and Ardrossan, the poorer parts of Ayrshire. They tended to be multiparas, some having had five or six pregnancies, little antenatal care, and practising no form of contraception mainly for religious reasons.

Once, in the middle of the night when I was at the labour ward, a GP rang me from Ayr and asked me how to put on forceps. I asked him for some details about the problem, which was in the hospital in Ayr. It did appear she required a forceps delivery and I offered the services of the flying squad because I did not think it appropriate for a doctor with no previous experience to be trying this manoeuvre. He would not accept this and insisted I explain how he performed this technique. It was difficult for a house officer to argue with a senior doctor, albeit he was a GP. I never heard the outcome of this, but when it went into the report in the morning, the chief quickly called me in to elaborate further. He was furious and stormed off to do battle with the GP.

The other consultant was Dr Forsyth. Not so flamboyant, but a nice boss also. One day on the way to an emergency with him, he told me an interesting story. He had been a doctor in the navy during the war and was on a destroyer anchored at Gibraltar. The Commander-in-Chief Mediterranean at that time was the renowned Admiral Andrew Cunningham. On this particular day the Admiral's barge was seen approaching the destroyer and there was panic onboard as no officers seem to have been onboard except Forsyth (Robbie Robertson was not there on this occasion!). He organised the necessary party with bosun's pipe to meet the Admiral when he came onboard. "Haven't I met you before in Edinburgh, doctor?" the Admiral asked, going on to add, "in the anatomy department I think?"

"Yes sir, that is exactly right," replied Forsyth.

Now this Admiral must have met dozens of people every day of his life so this was a superb feat of memory very few could hope to equal. One of the text books in anatomy was written by Prof. Cunningham who I presume was a relation to the admiral, hence his presence in the anatomy department at Edinburgh.

As the end of my six months at the Ayrshire Central Hospital approached, so did the promised caesarean section. Dr de Soldenoff appeared as I started to scrub up in theatre. The patient had had her cocktail so was just rousable and no more. She was being wheeled in and transferred to the operating table. "Just start when you are ready, I will be along in a short time," and with that the boss left theatre.

I knew the theatre sister very well, having worked with her for almost six months. Standing on the opposite side of the patient from her I said, "I am not keen to start until Dr de Soldenoff comes back."

"He will expect you to be well on with it when he returns," she replied.

I therefore proceeded to infiltrate the tissues with local anaesthetic meanwhile carrying on this conversation with sister. De Soldenoff popped into theatre at this stage, glanced at the patient's abdomen, told me to carry on and popped out again. I made my incision and worked my way down until the pregnant uterus appeared. At this stage – the most crucial – I refused to start the next cut and said so to sister, probably adding things like "this is my first time," "I don't really have a clue," etc. With that, the great man appeared, scrubbed up and came to assist me. Under his eye, I finished off the job, feeling extremely proud of myself.

Later that day, I went to see *my* patient. She was fine, and said, "I did not feel a thing, but I heard you speaking to sister!"

I had by this time made the big decision; I would go into general practice. Dr Peter Peterson, in practice at this time in Lerwick, asked me if I would come back to Shetland and become his trainee. This was a splendid offer because it saved me looking for a trainee job elsewhere and allowed me to come back home. I had decided when I did medicine that I was probably condemning myself to a life of exile. After all, there were so few practices in Shetland. However, I had grave doubts about taking up his offer. The reason was simply that I had been brought up in

Lerwick and knew so many people that I felt it might be embarrassing for some of the patients and, furthermore, I was afraid of expectations from some that they would be on a good wicket, particularly with sickness benefit.

Peter was very persistent and eventually I agreed to give it a try, provided that if I found it difficult to practice in Lerwick he would let me terminate my contract early. Normally the term of the traineeship was a year but I wanted an option to get out after a month. As it so happened, I never at any time during the year had a patient make any attempt to use previous acquaintance.

As I stepped off the boat to start my traineeship I was met by my uncle, John Johnston, who was Clerk to the Executive Council. This body dealt with all the general practices in Shetland. This included payments, doctors' tied houses, appointments to practices and a real helping hand for all the general practitioners.

There was a problem. Unst had been vacant awaiting the arrival of a new doctor who had been appointed. In the interim, locums had been covering the practice and the last one was just about to finish. That left two weeks until Dr Dunnet arrived. Would I go immediately to Unst for two weeks? I said I would but would have to clear it with Dr Peterson as he expected me to start with him.

Peter agreed I would start two weeks later and so I was on the *Earl of Zetland* heading for Unst at 8am the following day. The Executive Council had hired an old Land Rover for the various locums and when I landed off the flit boat at Uyeasound, there was the Land Rover and the locum to meet me. Imagine my surprise to find the locum was John Coutts, who had been in my year at Aberdeen. John had Trondra connections but lived in Aberdeen. I remember he was related to Willie Peterson, the auctioneer, possibly a cousin. John ended up in Tasmania where I presume he still is.

John took me up to the doctor's house, Hillsgarth, in Baltasound, which was totally empty except for one room at the back of the house which was the surgery. It was a bleak establishment, made worse by the dark, wet, windy evening when I got there. This was not improved when John very seriously said the place was haunted. When I laughed at him, he insisted there were strange noises in the surgery. I was surprised that such a down-to-earth fellow as John Coutts could believe in ghosts, at the same time a little relieved to know I would not be staying in the house. Digs had been arranged at Halligarth with Lorna Saxby and so we made our way there to a nice warm kitchen and an excellent supper. Lorna was a good cook and I enjoyed my two weeks digs there. I have a feeling there was no mains electricity though Stephen Saxby had a generator of sorts. Paraffin lamps were required upstairs and this took me back to country holidays in the past, especially the smell of burning paraffin.

I subsequently heard the noise in the surgery, and alone in there in the evening it started to prey a little on my mind too. I called in a witness and he discovered a bird in the lum. That was the ghost exorcised.

The kitchen at Hillsgarth had an Aga but it was the worst Aga I ever came across. It never gave off any heat and just heated the water but no more. During the day a woman, Rosie Petrie, appeared in the kitchen. She had been employed by the previous doctor. Being on a temporary basis, none of this concerned me and the two weeks flew by. Dr Dunnet was due on the Friday afternoon *Earl* and it was arranged for him to disembark at Uyeasound rather than suffer another hour going round to Baltasound. I set off for Uyeasound to meet him, in the dark with a gale and pouring rain. Half way to Uyeasound the Land Rover got a puncture. I was a bit short of time and unacquainted with the wheel changing on this type of vehicle so it was wet, dirty and flustered that I arrived at Sandison's shop at Uyeasound.

I picked up the new doctor, took him to Hillsgarth, showed him the surgery and took him to his digs. He would go down to the pier at Baltasound later when his car had been off-loaded from the *Earl*, and that was me finished. I foolishly went up to Saxa Vord to the Sergeant's Mess with Stephen Saxby and forgot

I was to be on the *Earl* at 6am for Lerwick. Even the hospitality of Captain Willie Sinclair on the bridge of the *Earl* next day did little to help the gastric unease. It was a typical bad weather day and I survived intact but only just.

One of the things I felt most strongly about in later years was the breakfast system on board the *Earl* during the summer months when the 'trippers' were on board. The vessel depended on the isles folk for its existence but we became second class passengers during the summer. This was nothing to do with the crew who were helpful, kind and courteous at all times, but somebody in Aberdeen had laid down company policy. To travel on the *Earl* leaving Baltasound at 6am meant an early start of 4am what with last minute packing, etc. to do. This meant that about seven o'clock the smell of fried bacon on the deck produced the well known Pavlovian response. However, tourists who had only got out of bed at 7.30 had priority for the first sitting at breakfast at 8am. The local people had to wait for the second sitting somewhere nearer 9am.

As I stood on the deck Captain Sinclair came down from the bridge. "Are you not going in for breakfast?" he asked.

I was becoming hypoglycaemic and therefore on a short fuse by this time. When I explained the situation he immediately invited me in to sit at the officer's table. The officers consisted of captain, mate and chief, who were much better company than the tourists who filled the dining room. I never had to wait for second sitting after that and never forgot Willie's kindness. It was typical of the kindness and consideration which pervaded the entire *Earl* in those days.

The wings of the bridge of the *Earl* allowed a few people to stand immediately behind the main bridge. Willie would engage these tourists in conversation and often invite some onto the bridge proper. These tourists sometimes asked the most ridiculous questions. One English lady asked the mate if he was ever scared in bad weather. People who knew Willie Sinclair will remember he had a florid complexion. Willie was in the wheelhouse at the time when the mate replied, "Only if I see the skipper's face go pale."

Shortly after I started with Peter Peterson, Maureen moved back to the 'Annexe' to work. She had spent some time working there previously and our earliest encounter had been at that time when she had offered to help me pull a boat up at the Craigie Stane. I declined her offer, in fact would rather have burst than to have had a woman help me.

Anyway, we got married on 1st March, 1960, and managed to rent 'Willowbrae' in Charlotte Street. This was a funny little house but very convenient in every way.

I was very lucky to be able to work with Peter. He had a wealth of experience, having spent many years in Yell. He had a great sense of humour and was very dedicated to his job. Peter was just as keen as I was on boats, fishing and the freedom to indulge in them, something he had little chance to do, being always on call in a single-handed practice. After a few weeks I was promoted to do an equal share of the work. Peter made out a timetable over a fortnight so that I had exactly the same time off as he did. This was in the days when trainees got little time off. Most principals used their trainees to their own advantage, but not Peter.

This year was instructive for me and I learned all sorts of new mixtures, ointments, etc., many of them being Peter's own recipes. In those days there was much less of the proprietary medicines, linctuses, etc. which later became the norm. His favourite antibiotic was Chloromycetin, which even then was beginning to go into disfavour. However, he used it in very short treatments of four days and I fell in with this routine. Later I used it only for very specific conditions, becoming more afraid of its side effects. Chloromycetin came as a syrup, but the usual form was as a capsule.

Being fairly recently taught forensic medicine, I tended to see flamingos sometimes when they were only scories. An illustration of this took place in Sandwick. Peter's practice, like Dr Cadenhead's practice, had quite a few patients in Sandwick and Cunningsburgh. The practice was reasonably small and therefore, being paid per capita, it meant having patients outwith Lerwick. The patient had been seen the day before by Peter and given Chloromycetin capsules for a chest infection. The next day, he collapsed after eating a sandwich which his wife had prepared and I was called to see him. He had complained when eating the sandwich of its very bitter taste. Man and wife did not get on together and alarm bells rang in my head - strychnine! However, no court case was to develop as I discovered by further questioning of his wife. She had opened the Chloromycetin capsule and poured its contents into his sandwich. It was in a capsule to be swallowed whole precisely because of its bitter taste.

During my year with Peter, a request came through asking if one of us would go to Levenwick as Dr John Hamilton had become ill and there was nobody to look after the practice. I was delegated and set off for Levenwick in my A30. Over the next few days I was to discover that a heater in a car was not a luxury item as I had previously thought and later on I had a rather inefficient type fitted. At least it helped to keep the windscreen clear if doing little for my feet and legs. The first night I was there, there was an extremely heavy snowfall. Everything was blocked next morning, the snow being right to the roof of the garage.

One of the first duties when I arrived was to go upstairs and examine Dr Hamilton, who was in bed. I was apprehensive about this as I knew John Hamilton as one of the most senior practitioners in Shetland. His tall, rather severe appearance, complete with deerstalker hat and rimless spectacles, and reputation of being an authoritarian figure did not help. Even worse, I knew he was a bit old fashioned and did not believe in antibiotics. I was between the devil and the deep sea for Mrs Hamilton ruled the roost and in no way could you argue the point with that lady. So I did as she ordered and went up to see John.

He was very pleasant and grateful for my presence to look after the practice. I examined him and he had a chest infection. He then asked me what he should take. I suggested he should have an antibiotic and he agreed without argument. "What one would you suggest?" he enquired. We agreed on penicillin and an expectorant mixture, the latter being his own mixture which he preferred. I took the medicines up to him, but whether he took my penicillin or not, I don't know. He got better anyway, and I like to think he did.

In those days snow clearing was a bit primitive and often required manual digging to help the snow clearing vehicle. So there being no emergencies for the next three days, I read books from the excellent selection available. Mrs Hamilton was a superb cook and the food was excellent. It was difficult under the circumstances to always do the right thing, be in the right place and generally try to avoid stepping on Mrs Hamilton's toes. They had a very set routine and it was foreign to me. They were very kind and hospitable really and I survived the few days until I could get out, and shortly afterwards John took over the practice again and I reported to Peter Peterson.

A month or two later John Hamilton acquired a trainee, my great friend from student days, Martin Lees. This was a great social asset for Maureen and me as Martin would come up to Willowbrae each week on his half-day. It did not take long for Martin to forget the cares of the previous week before he was rolling round laughing with the tears running down his cheeks.

It had been relatively easy for me to spend a few days in Levenwick but Martin had a difficult path to tread as he also lived with Dr John and Mrs Hamilton. The routine was sacred. Each evening at a certain time Martin was told he had to use the bathroom as John used it at a set time before Mrs Hamilton, then it was bedtime. Martin had no option but to comply. Martin was the first to say how kind and good they were to him at Gord, but it was rather restrictive.

To eke out the practice income, Peter did all the dental anaesthetics and did them well. I was thus introduced to the school dentist, John Allan, and to Bruce Laurenson in Mounthooly Street. I did not really require an introduction to the latter as he had been my dentist when I was in Lerwick. Bruce was a great character, fanatically keen on the lifeboat and sailing, a very good dentist, but no business manager. The first time I went to give him dental anaesthetics, Peter told me to make sure he paid me. I said I could not possibly ask for the money as my folk never had a bill for any treatment I had had from him in the past. The way out of this difficulty was to ask at the end of the session for the little black book. In this anaesthetic fees were entered and this produced not only the book, but the required number of pounds, taken from a pile of money which lay on his desk in the surgery.

After I went to Unst I heard a story about Bruce. The minister in Unst sometime previously was fond of a dram and it was difficult to get one in Unst, the isle being dry with no retail outlets. The answer lay in dental appointments in Lerwick with Bruce, who was very careful and thorough but very slow. This, of course, suited the minister well as it meant infinite trips to Lerwick. Bruce was making a denture for the minister and eventually it was fitted. On the next Sunday the minister asked one of the elders after the service what they thought about his sermon. "It was all right minister, except when you said the letter 'S', when you seemed to whistle through your new teeth. It was very pronounced every time you said 'Jesus Christ'."

"Goodness gracious," said the minister, "I will have to go down to Lerwick again and see Mr Laurenson."

On being asked what the trouble was the minister explained about the whistling, but did not refer to Jesus. Bruce took the teeth over to his sink in the corner and filed a bit off them and handed them back to the minister. "Try that," he said.

He was busy washing his hands with his back to the minister when he heard, "Jesus Christ, Jesus Christ."

Bruce whirled around and said, "What the bloody hell is wrong with them now?"

Maureen was left sitting for a long while one day in Bruce's dental chair. The view from the chair was over the Market Cross and she sat patiently with these things that are put in your mouth for various reasons. Bruce seemed to be a long time in the laboratory which was behind the surgery on the way out, when she suddenly spotted him making towards the breakwater for a lifeboat alert!

One of Peter's quotations I retained for the rest of my working life: "If you get called to a sick child and you have made sure it does not have meningitis or appendicitis, you can go home to your bed again." A simplification perhaps, but a good enough basic rule.

Peter was full of yarns, mainly about his time in Yell. When he'd arrived to take over from Dr Gilchrist, at the end of the hand-over Gilchrist had handed him something and said, "You had better have this."

When Peter looked, it was a small revolver. "What for?" asked Peter.

"The dogs," Gilchrist replied. Apparently he was terrified of dogs.

During the war Peter had been called one day to a croft which lay on the side of a hill. There was no road so it meant walking to the bottom of a valley and climbing the other side. When Peter entered the croft the old couple were sitting one each side of the fire with gas masks on. When Peter managed to persuade them to take them off the old man said, "We smelled a bad smell and thought the Germans had dropped gas, so we thought we would better send for the doctor"! Some folk seem to think doctors are immune to everything, even poison gas.

There was one neurotic lady in the practice who attended surgery two or three times a week with a new illness each time. We had more or less given up trying to cure her complaints or even to try and PLEASE her. She was never even mildly grateful for anything which we tried to do. One Friday surgery which I took she appeared again with a new set of complaints and, after listening for some time, I had to try and sort the chiff from the chaff if that was possible, and then to accede to her demand which was sure to come for some medicine to cure her. By this stage I had stopped writing up her notes fully and I gave her a prescription for a new proprietary preparation.

On Saturday morning Peter was taking the surgery and I was off. The phone rang and this was Peter. The same patient was at the surgery yet again but this time she was pleased because the tablet which I had prescribed the day before was the first tablet she had ever had which had done her some good. "What did you give her?" Peter asked. "There is no note of it in her notes."

"I can't remember what her complaint was, let alone the tablet," I replied.

"Never mind, she has brought two tablets with her so you can take one to two chemists on Monday and I will take the other one to the other two pharmacies."

We both spent about an hour on Monday but no chemist in Lerwick could recognise the tablet. Peter had the pleasure of breaking the news at the next surgery. She promptly left the practice and transferred her custom to one of the other practices in the town. I often told Peter that if I had done nothing else in my year with him, I had at least relieved him of this impossible patient.

One female patient had some infertility problems and was one of those people who talk loudly in public about their medical problems. She consulted me about her problem and I was very amused to hear via the town gossip some time later that, "If it had no been for Dr Robertson I widna be pregnant the day."

Fortunately the General Medical Council never heard what she was telling everybody!

My year as a trainee was drawing to an end. Peter had a proposition for me. If we could expand the practice in some way there would be a modest living for two, especially if we could divide up the large house he lived in, and which had the surgery in the basement, into two flats. He was offering me a partnership and what an offer to a young doctor at that time. Often you had to wait a long time to get into partnership and then only to discover the doctors did not get along too well. Here the relationship was good and even though it entailed a fairly low salary, being young and optimistic I was sure we could build the practice up. There were all sorts of things to be looked into and at the end of my year a locum job for three weeks cropped up in Voe for Dr David Porter.

I took over the Voe practice and David Porter set off for Sumburgh only to return, that day and the following one. He eventually got out on the third day. We were asked to look after Bill and this was our introduction to Staffordshire bull terriers. We eventually acquired one for ourselves and now have the fourth. They are very loyal dogs with great personality and often no fear. Each one we have known has its own personality and all are different in so many ways.

The first evening surgery at Voe a man appeared and asked for tablets for a lady somewhere in the Vidlin area. There was a triple reference system in the practice which I had been shown but on going through the three books I could not find the diagnosis, or the regular prescription. However, the messenger offered the diagnosis in lay terms and I gave him the appropriate tablets.

The following morning I began to have doubts about the wisdom of prescribing on such vague information and told Maureen I was going to nip across and check the accuracy of the prescription. I set out with Bill, who liked to go in the car, after morning surgery and eventually found my way to the end of the road at Sweening. My destination was Sandwick and on asking at Sweening was told it was around the corner further out the voe. I set off in heavy showers, taking the dog with me for the walk. On reaching the 'corner' there was another headland beyond but no house, so I expected to find it when I reached the next inlet. At this point Bill set off after a rabbit and I had to retrace some ground to find him and then put him on a lead. I walked on and on and began to have doubts about the veracity of my directions. Eventually, round another corner and there was a thatched roof house with the lum reeking.

I received a royal welcome, my coat was taken to the fire – an open peat fire with crook – and before I knew where I was tea, bread, bannocks and boiled eggs appeared before me. The tablets had still not arrived but were the right ones. All the latest news on the radio had to be discussed and it was well into the afternoon before I could get away again. By the time I got back to Voe a full scale emergency was almost about to be initiated.

I enjoyed my three weeks at Voe, mainly because the patients were fine folk. I preferred working in a country practice to working in the town.

Unst was going to be vacant. Now that news upset the applecart. It might be years before another practice was available but I was half committed to Dr Peterson and I would not have let him down when he had set his heart on a partnership. So the first thing to do was to go and discuss it with him.

He was not in when I called. I sat and spoke to Ina until he returned. I was keen on Unst but felt committed to the Lerwick venture so was a bit uncomfortable about broaching the subject. Peter came in and said, "Hello, I expect you are wanting to apply for Unst?"

That made it easy for me to say I came to discuss it.

"Apply for it, and I will give you my support. You will be much more secure there than in the proposed partnership here."

Having cleared the air on that issue, Peter brought up another, taking out teeth. This was a skill I did not have but would be expected to possess. I would be sure to be asked at any interview for an island practice. John Allan, the school dentist at the time, kindly agreed to let me take out some teeth to become familiar with the instruments and the technique. He also showed me how to do an inferior dental nerve block with local anaesthetic. I was therefore armed, be it ever so lightly, for the dental question should I get an interview.

I then went back to Voe to continue the locum and by sheer coincidence I received a call to Vidlin a few days later which put temptation in front of me. The patient was W.R.T. Hamilton and he was chairman of the Executive Council. Having examined him and advised him to stay inside for the next few days and to take an antibiotic which I would send, he asked me if I was going to apply for Unst. I replied I had already done so. "I would support your application at the meeting in two days time."

To have the chairman's support was very important but the weather was bitterly cold with a north wind which went right through you and I decided I would have to sacrifice his attendance at the meeting in view of his complaint. Furthermore, I had already advised him in that direction. It might have been more disappointing to lose this support but he then went on to say, "I will make my views known to the Clerk of the Executive Council on the interview day even though I cannot attend." It was a very nice gesture which I appreciated very much.

The candidates for interview had been short listed to three and the best rival as far as I was concerned was a Dr Alex Laing. I was very pleased later to see him appointed to the Walls practice which became vacant not very long afterwards. Little did I know that in a few short years I would be coming down from Unst to attend his funeral. Alex was a great loss to the west side and to medicine in Shetland.

Eventually I was called back into the Executive Council and told I had been appointed to Unst. They would be glad if I could take up the job on 17th December, 1960, as Dr Dunnet was hoping to leave that day.

Chapter 8

Unst

IF the weather had been an augury I would never have gone to Unst. 17th December, 1960, was like so many days at that time of the year in Shetland, grey, windy, cold and wet. It was dark when we sailed on the *Earl* at 8am and it was dark when we arrived in Uyeasound about 4pm. Going ashore in the flit boat, sitting on top of the mail, made for a very damp arrival. It was even worse for Maureen who was now very pregnant.

Where was Dr Dunnet whom I had struggled to meet exactly a year earlier at the same place? All we could do was file aboard the bus and be deposited at Hillsgarth, the doctor's house in Baltasound which I was briefly familiar with from the year before.

What a depressing welcome. The house was empty, dark and cold, apart from a light in the kitchen at the back. Here we found the departing doctor. He made some feeble excuse when I said we expected a taxi or some vehicle to meet us, not actually expressing my thoughts that he could have done it himself. He was just about to leave and had actually done so when he reappeared muttering about a razor blade he had left in the bathroom. That was the only thing he did leave or nearly leave.

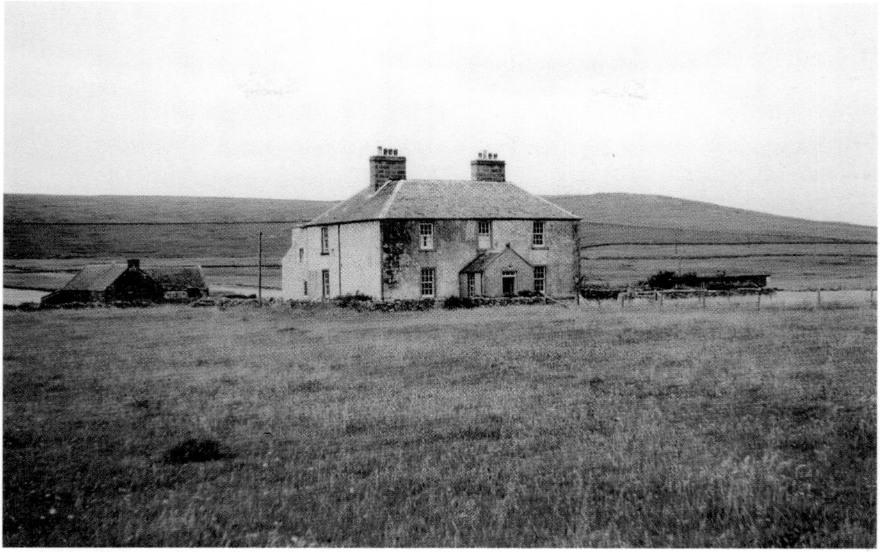

Hillsgarth, Unst – the doctor's house in 1960.

The Aga was out, there was not one lump of fuel in the coal cellar, the bulbs in the ceiling lamp holders had been removed apart from in a few essential rooms.

Later we received what little furniture and fittings we possessed when the *Earl* reached Baltasound. Our first meal was cooked in our only pan on an upturned electric fire. We ate off an orange box, got the bed assembled and made up and probably went to bed with our socks and hats on.

The house was a well built two-storey ex-manse, very square with big rooms and high ceilings, very elegant, but very difficult to heat, and not improved by stone flags in the hall right through the house and in the kitchen. It was a week before we could get fuel for the Aga and when we did it was warm to touch but that was all. The decoration was war-time distemper in drab greens and beige. Although it all sounds depressing, we were not in the slightest bit put off, being young and having been handed a practice to run and develop, the newness and interest neutralised the effect of the house.

The house layout was simple, four rooms in a square with a large hall running between and a front porch. The room on the left as you came in was the waiting room, quite empty apart from some chairs. The room at the back on the right was the surgery with a cupboard in the hall as extra drug storage. The rest of the drugs were stored in a cupboard alongside the 'haunted' fireplace. These facilities appeared adequate at the time but nowadays would appear quite Dickensian.

There were some old agricultural buildings at the back of the house, some sheds, a garage and a large walled garden which had been a showpiece some years earlier but had now gone back to a jungle.

Surgery times were 9.30 to 10.30 each morning, including Saturday, with sick parade twice a week at RAF Saxa Vord. This sick parade was then followed by a branch surgery for people in Haroldswick. An afternoon surgery was held in the vestry of the kirk at Uyeasound on Wednesday. During my time the only thing I altered was to introduce an antenatal clinic on Tuesday mornings. The essential surgery fittings, i.e. an old desk and an examination couch, I purchased from my predecessor. I started off with my second-hand faithful old friend, the Austin A30, later going up market, or down as you think fit, to a new A35 van.

That first Christmas day in Unst was not very exciting, apart from the appearance of a man on a bike at 9 o'clock on the 25th. When I got out of bed to see what he wanted, he said he had come to the surgery for a consultation. He had cycled from Haroldswick (about five miles). I was not very keen to see him on that particular day and did not want to set a precedent for other so-called holidays but under the circumstances agreed to see him. He had a cold! To be fair, this one man tended to push his luck, but he was the only one and I never had any further problems of that kind.

I had decided I would have to set the rules and stick to them. Otherwise a single-handed doctor in a rural practice could be running all over the place without reason as well as trying to establish some sort of 'free time' for himself. Free time could of

Tiverton Library

Phone enquiries: 0345 155 1001
www.devonlibraries.org.uk

Interested in a Beginner's Computing Course?
Ask us for more information.

Renewed Items 23/07/2019 10:34
XXXXXXXXXX3071

Item Title	Due Date
Very short history of Western thought	13/08/2019

course never be guaranteed when on call every day but a true emergency was something no doctor objected to. The first of these turned up at the back door of the house about 2am. There was a dance on somewhere in the island with the casualty, like everybody else, having a half bottle in the back pocket of his trousers. Somehow he had landed on his backside with catastrophic results. He had lost his whisky, ruined a pair of trousers, and badly lacerated his posterior. He lay quietly on the couch while I anaesthetised the area (there was no need for sterilisation) then stitched it up.

The woman who had been employed by previous doctors as a maid turned up but there was nothing for her to do and she, poor soul, did not inspire much cheer so we decided to do without her. Later we were very relieved we had taken this unpleasant path because we struck pure gold.

This barn of a house, with five bedrooms upstairs and a bathroom, was slowly improved and made more comfortable, partly through our own efforts but also through diplomatic negotiations with the Executive Council. Their clerk of works was Davy Fotheringham and he was always sympathetic and helpful. They agreed to take up the flagstones and lay composite floors of concrete and sawdust mixture in the kitchen and the hallway, covered with hardboard. This eliminated the eternal dust of these surfaces and gave slightly better insulation. We eventually got rid of the Aga, substituting a solid fuel Rayburn, and much later on solid fuel central heating was installed. The former was later converted to oil. The latter was not much used as it required the full-time employment of a stoker as well as devouring fuel at a greedy rate.

Maureen's sister, Olive, came over from Donegal to stay with us and single-handedly painted and papered the entire house. It was a mammoth task which occupied her for many months. At the end of eighteen years, when we left the house, it was a great wrench. It had become a superb home for us with plenty of space which we had gradually furnished over the years.

The decision to build a surgery, dispensary and waiting room on the side of the house was made by the Executive Council after a few years. This was a most welcome addition (a) because the existing facilities were inadequate and (b) because it gave us the house to ourselves. Patients no longer came in our front door and sat in the house but had a means of approach to the new surgery round the side of it. The heating of the house improved once the front door was not continuously being opened and closed during the morning surgery.

The work on the extension proved difficult in one aspect. The new surgery required a door through from the original surgery. This was taken out where a window was but a new window had to be knocked out in the back of the room to replace it. The wall was very thick, built of large blocks of stone keyed into one another. When it was completed it gave us another room, albeit with a passage through it. There is now a much more extensive and new surgery development built beyond the house.

I had a contract with Royal Air Force Strike Command to provide medical services at the radar station, RAF Saxa Vord. The contract helped with the income of the practice which was just on the edge of inducement practice size. Inducement practices were decided by size of population and therefore income. I applied but was not accepted on the grounds that the practice was not socially deprived.

Having arrived in Unst just before Christmas, there was more disruption when on Hogmanay Maureen started to 'niggle'. She therefore took the opportunity of the *Earl* that day to go down to Lerwick.

In the middle of the night a few days later I was woken by the phone. "Peter here."

"Yes, what news Peter?"

"Did I ever tell you about the bike which had no saddle bag and pump?" was the reply.

I did not catch on and when I was anxious for news thought little of Peter's phone call in the middle of the night to tell me jokes I did not understand. After he had repeated this he explained Maureen had had a girl and both were fine. A saddle bag did arrive eventually and then another without.

As the family grew it became more difficult for Maureen to look after them, the house and the phone. The phone in particular could be difficult in the middle of bathing a baby or

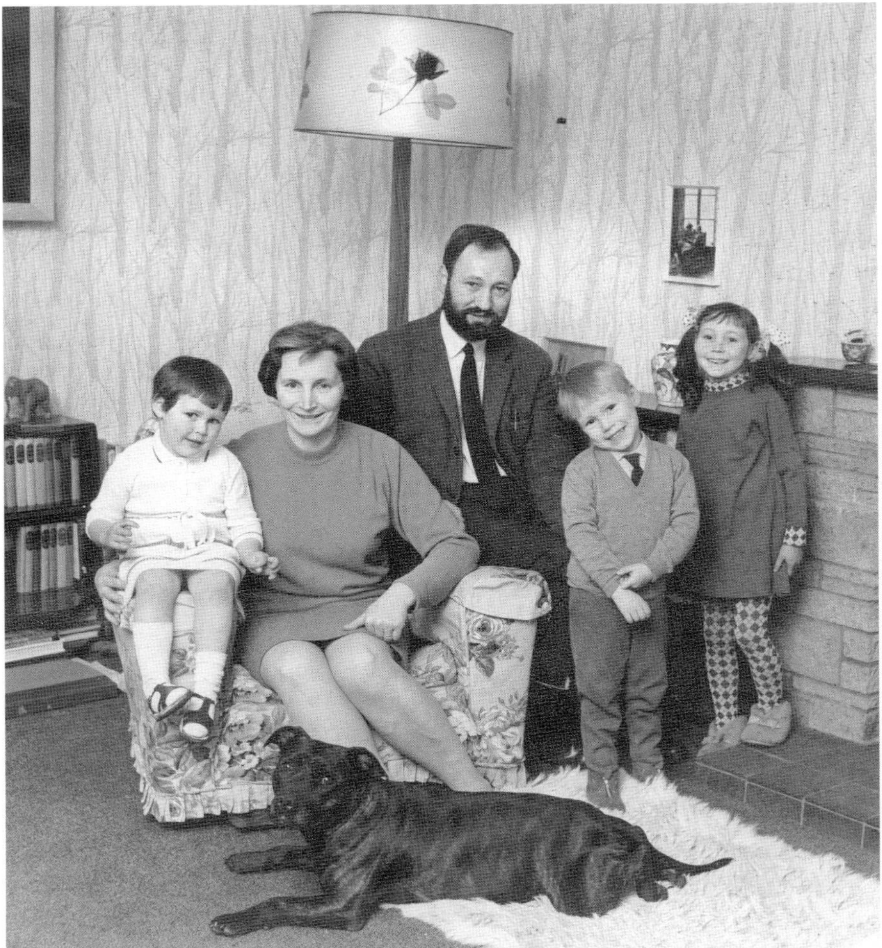

The family with Rasmie the dog at Hillsgarth, Unst: Jane, Maureen, the author, John, Susan. *Photo: Dennis Coutts*

rolling out pastry, or even just to leave small children unattended when answering it. It also required to be answered 24 hours a day. It was a considerable commitment which all doctors' wives undertook without recompense or recognition in those days.

The one great asset as far as the phone was concerned was the manual telephone exchange at Baltasound. It was thanks to Gilda Thomson who manned the exchange that we could get away from the phone. Provided we went somewhere near another phone, a ring to Gilda to say where I would be was sufficient. If a call came though the exchange, Gilda would ask if it was urgent. If it was, she then phoned me at the substitute number. Every Sunday in the summer in those days seemed to be beautifully warm and sunny so that we could take the children and go to the Skaw beach. The Sinclairs at Skaw were always most willing to come down to the beach if I was required. Gilda acted as my 'ansaphone' long before they materialised. It was a service to me and the community for which we were all truly grateful.

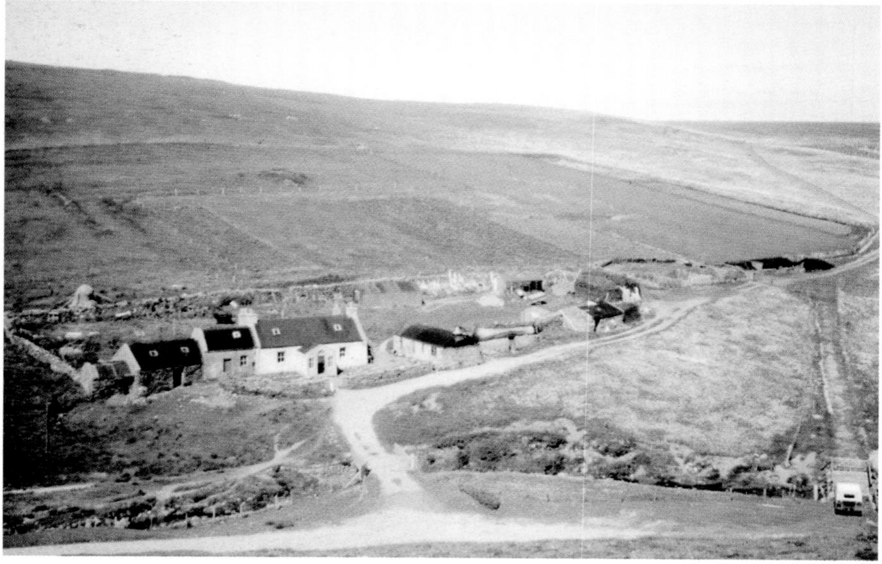

Skaw – the most northerly house in Great Britain.

There was a bright light on the horizon as far as the domestic situation was concerned. This was in the form of Beth Inkster, who came to work for us and as there was plenty of room in the house and, transport not what it is now, stayed in during the week, going home at week ends. Now we did have some freedom to go out in the evening knowing the children and the phone were in the capable hands of Beth.

What a treasure Beth proved to be. She was discreet, one of the most important aspects of employment in a doctor's house, reliable, full of common sense and quiet, but if she did speak it was of some relevance. She had the bedroom which looked east across Baltasound and when all the excitement was in progress the day Springfield Hotel went on fire, Beth was heard to say quietly, "I thought I saw a lot of smoke from there when I got up." She had never mentioned it until then.

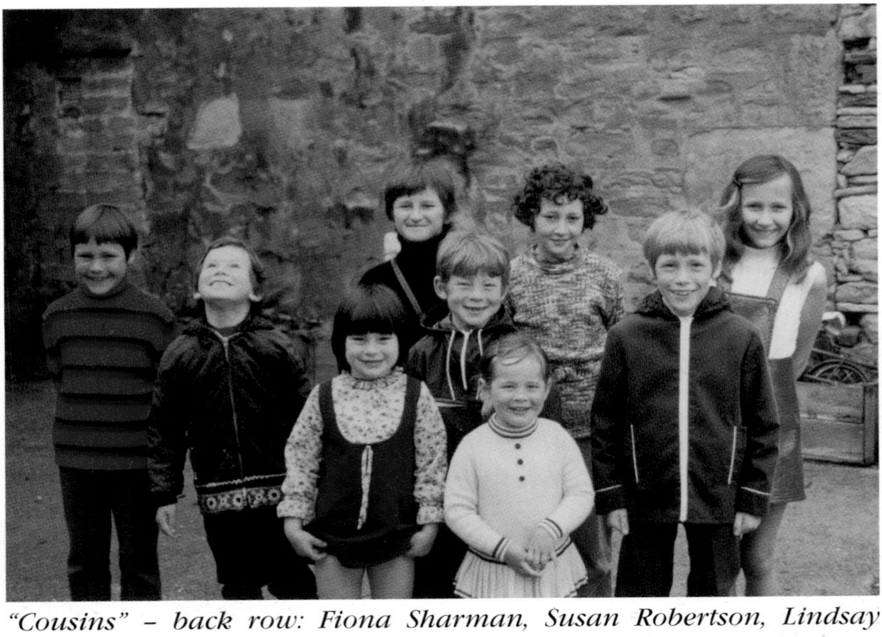

"Cousins" – back row: Fiona Sharman, Susan Robertson, Lindsay Sharman. Middle: Jane Robertson, Graham Sharman, Michael Moore, John Robertson. Front: Nicola Moore, Jennifer Moore.

Chapter 9

Back to the RAF

SHORTLY after I arrived in Unst there was a terrific gale. The house had two central chimney stacks built through both floors. At the height of the gale a glass-fronted cupboard alongside the chimney stack downstairs was vibrating to such an extent it could be seen from light reflection in the glass quite easily. The noise was tremendous and the carpet in the front room was floating, giving an unreal feel when walking over it. These were phenomena we were to experience many times in the years to come.

On this particular night I received a mysterious phone call in the evening from Saxa Vord. Could I please attend as there had been an accident? No more details were given nor did it sound likely I would get them if I had asked. On arrival at the station sick quarters I was met by the orderly officer. He enquired if there was a room where he could speak to me privately. On going into the consulting room he said there had been an accident with the radar scanner but it was highly confidential. I was sworn to secrecy. Two airmen had been near, were physically unhurt, but a little shocked. I saw them, dealt with their fright as best I could and drove home.

At the morning surgery next day the first patient was an old lady from Haroldswick. Most consultations were held after an introductory preamble, usually concerning the weather and perhaps an enquiry as to how I was keeping. She opened with, "Awful night last night, wasn't it?"

"Yes," I replied, "one of the worst gales I have experienced."

"The scanner blew down," was her next remark. I was a bit taken aback for a moment to think this ordinary Shetland woman knew this secret and furthermore was speaking about it quite openly. It was a little naive of me not to have given the scanner incident some thought and to have realised it was like removing the Town Hall in Lerwick overnight. As it dominated the skyline in Lerwick, so the scanner on the top of Saxa Vord hill did in Unst.

That very same day a Russian 'trawler' with a great array of aerials and antennae came into Burrafirth, which lies immediately below Saxa Vord, and lay there for the next day or so in spite of my sealed lips. It was following this that a huge radome was erected from fibreglass panels to protect the 22-ton radar scanner from future gales.

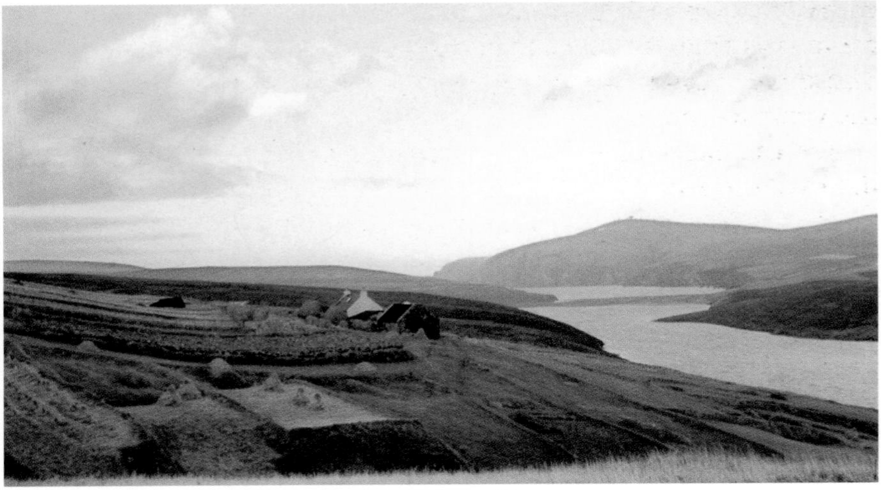

Well-cultivated Pettister, Unst, in the 1960s.

It was at Saxa Vord that the record wind speed was recorded, with a gust of 177mph. I was driving along the road at Ordale on the south side of Baltasound about that time. There was no ditch, luckily, at that part of the road as I suddenly found myself driving on the grass. Violent correction brought the van back on to the road and I continued on my way. It was only later, when I heard about the gust, that I realised it coincided with my off-road driving.

The gales at that time seemed to be from the south-east. They blew for days on end with complete cessation of all transport in and out of Unst. No *Earl of Zetland* for a week perhaps, began to make its effect felt on the perishables in the shops. In these days before supermarkets and inter-island roll-on-roll-off ferries, Unst was well served by shops. The biggest was Sandison's at Skibhoul where anything from a needle to an anchor or a cabbage could be obtained. It, like all the shops, was a counter shop. It took time to gather a shopping list together at the counter, the assistant walking many miles in a day, back and fore, collecting the order on the counter. Bread was baked next door daily, with meat available in the shop as well as at 'Bertie Butcher's' shop nearby. A number, if not most people, walked to the shop which was a meeting place for all the latest news. No urgency in being served lengthened the discourse and offered more chance of meeting more customers. It was only when I was not in Unst I discovered how convenient it had been to get a pick handle, some screw nails, clothes, a pound of tea, meat and a gallon of paraffin all in one shop, instead of having to go here for this and somewhere else for that.

Nessie Henderson had a small shop in Baltasound; nearby Harry Henderson had a bigger establishment with a variety of goods; there was a shop at Virse in Norwick; another Sandison shop in Haroldswick; and a shop near Burrafirth owned by Alex Priest. There were two shops in Uyeasound, one at the pier owned by Sandisons, and the other, run by J.J. Hunter and Harold Sutherland under the name of Humprey's, at the east side. This latter shop was a virtual Aladdin's cave, normally referred to as

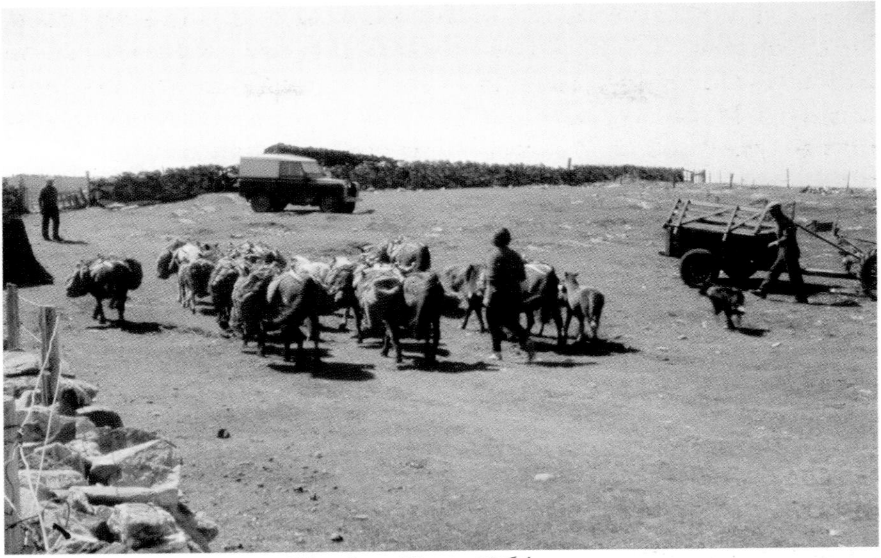

Flitting peats by pony, Westing, Unst, 1964.

'Harold's'. To say to Harold, I don't suppose you would have a such and such, was to ask a rhetorical question. RAF families later called it 'Harrods'.

People who worked at Saxa Vord had access to the NAAFI shop at the camp also. This shop produced a greater variety for those who could use it.

All the shops were 'dry'. A vote later made Unst wet. Officially, if any alcohol was required, it had to be taken in by the dozen from a wholesaler. This was the legal requirement but a constant stream of brown paper parcels came across from Greenbank in Yell, very often with the policeman on a Friday morning. This was the standard day of the police visit, when all unlicensed vehicles were immobilised or put out of sight. By lunch time the policeman was on the overland ferry back to Yell for another week. There was no crime anyway. A very occasional small theft pointed at the same one or two. In eighteen years I never locked my car or the house. Later, when the new surgery was built, I locked it up if I was absent for a period. The outside door, however, had to be left unlocked for prescriptions to be collected.

Drugs being sent throughout the island were dispersed with the school children. I made up the day's prescriptions, apart from those dispensed at surgery, and when all were ready I took them up to William John Thomson, the school canteen cook. He gave the items to the child who lived nearest the recipient. Only once was a bottle broken and very, very occasionally the drugs were forgotten in a schoolbag.

Some people thought this was a dangerous means of conveyance. They did not take into account the service this provided for all in a rural community nor the good common sense and awareness of duty all these children were endowed with. Admittedly, these were the days before the misuse of drugs became so prevalent. I had complete faith in the system and it never let me down.

Like all goods, my drugs came in once a week on Friday night with the *Earl*. They were then delivered by John Sutherland (Spragatup) on Friday night or Saturday morning. The drugs always came in tea chests packed with straw. Now it is cardboard boxes full of polystyrene shapes.

The value of this weekly consignment was considerable, even in those days. At Christmas I was rather annoyed to discover two slips of thin paper with a calendar provided by some drug company and overprinted by Paterson the wholesaler in Aberdeen with their Christmas greetings. I wrote to them and pointed out how mean I thought this was. An apologetic letter appeared with the next order and a small box of chocolates. Patersons stocked spirits and wine so I had expected at least a bottle of whisky!

One day, after I had been eight years in Unst, the Regional Medical Officer appeared at the surgery. He is a government employed doctor who, from a fair distance, keeps an eye on medical practices. He asked to see my Dangerous Drugs register. I had to admit I did not have such a thing, though it was statutory to keep one. He was very nice about it but warned me I had better have one next time he called. I obtained one the following week and thereafter kept it up to date, but I was never asked for it again.

Chapter 10

Spew

IF there was a delay with weather or a preparation I had run out of and needed before the next tea chest delivery, I phoned the chemist in Lerwick. I always dealt with Alex Campbell (Spew) at Porteous'. I dealt with him for two reasons: one - I knew him well; and two - he replied by letter. The letters were very clever epistles, full of amusing side stories and quotations. As a result, I still have the correspondence and make no excuses for repeating them here, word for word.

On the arrival of one of the children:

Dear Doc,

Most sincere congratulations and good wishes to you both. Of course you know this is the end of that refreshing eight hours sleep only Horlicks and a clear conscience can give. As William Shakespeare almost said in King Lear:

"How sharper than a thankless snake it is to have a toothless child."

Ingratiate though his daughters were, Keeler and Rice-Davies were yet to come ... even so, the ole king had his troubles.

Please accept this small package with our compliments.

Again, kindest regards to your goodself and the wee yin.

Yours most sincerely
Alexander M. Campbell.

On the non-appearance of an order:

Dear Doc,

Your justifiable concern over the delay in sending your order is easily understood, and I am sorry you have had the trouble of having to write specially about it. We are working at half strength. Everything happens at once, of course. As soon as I pick up a piece of wrapping paper the phone goes, or the butcher's apprentice over the way chooses that moment to do a little do-it-yourself amputation, they find a new way every time. This is intended as an explanation rather than an excuse. Not to grumble, you were quite right to enquire as you did. Incidentally the one assistant, now married, who could have come back and resumed where she left off is expecting a child so that's that.

Sorry for all this disjointed screed but the spirit of Up Helly Aa dies hard within me, unfortunately.

Cheerio for now anyway; don't hesitate to ask for any assistance at any time (isn't that phrased bloody horribly?) Sorry can't help it.

Ever Yours
Me, when God preserve
-- meantime anyway.

On sending Alex an old prescription presented by a patient asking for a repeat:

Dear Doc,

Missive received and understood (pardon haste but am hoping to get this away with the Earl tomorrow). Have you looked at the date though? 1937 migawd! What do these people expect - I think you were born then but little more. Honestly ...

Well I doubt it is no longer on the market under that name although there is no harm in trying, even so. Failing that here are the ingredients...

[A long prescription follows then, he continues the letter:]

Hope this will help but ring if not. Kind regards to Missus and family and again excuse speedo.

Yours sincerely
Alex

Dear Doc,

Unfortunately Droxalin got discontinued and off the market completely but we do have the tablets which come in 2/6d packets of 30. Any use? It is the only form they are made in (or it is I should say).

Had a memorable encounter a week last Tuesday with an old yet sprightly mariner of some eighty summers, who had come down from Whalsay to watch the regatta. This worthy presented himself at the trading post asking if we kept such a thing as Blue Ointment, which we did. He then rhetorically convinced himself by saying "You have it then," three times over, adding something about a peerie green falcon. He was deafer than hell, by the way, but for all his roaring was most indistinct in his speech. "Oh yes," was about all one could say, whereupon he again bellowed something I could not catch, about his peerie green falcon. All I could think was that it might be the name of one of the boats sailing that afternoon, though I had never heard of any such craft, the princely art of falconry hardly seemed to fit in with the Bonney Isle. Meantime he was off again about the Blue Ointment. "Could he have a look?"

The shop was crowded so I thought I had better take him out of earshot to make sure he really knew what the Hell he was doing – I wasn't quite happy about it all, and I was fully expecting him to follow with a query if they were any good for the crabs at the pitch of his voice. It once happened before though not with him.

Anyway while it was impossible to get him totally out of earshot (he could be heard at Hepworths I'll guarantee) the peerie green falcon ultimately resolved itself into a Peregrine Falcon. That much was clear, but little else made sense. He spoke as if everyone knew about his ornithological showpiece, time was passing so I asked him point blank if he was going to use it on the bird. He didn't answer directly but this did bring to light the bloody thing was stuffed!

To cut a long story short, the wretched thing had great sentimental value and I imagine it had been a family heirloom for so long it was literally crawling. As a young man in the first World War he had indeed been afflicted with the relevant pediculi and found "Hit cleared them aff lik dat. Blawdy good suff hit wiz." Having observed to his distress that the bird was alive with fleas, he thought it would be a good idea to anoint it with the mixture as before, especially as they seemed to be most numerous between its legs.

"Dat wye," he added sympathetically, "we'll shift da buggers aff the face o' da ert."

With self control I didn't know I had, I managed to flog him a 1/3d DDT puffer instead. It verily takes all sorts ...

Sincerely

Alex

Chapter 11

More military tales

STATION sick quarters at RAF Saxa Vord had a permanent staff of three: two airmen and a corporal in charge. Like all personnel at this station, they were posted there for eighteen months. The quality varied a lot but on the whole they were quite good at their job, as far as training and experience would allow. One of the nursing orderlies spent two tours of duty at Saxa Vord, fortunately for me he was the best of the many who circulated through the job.

'Maddie', as he was and is commonly known still lives in Shetland, but now in Lerwick. Malcolm Maddison, to give him his proper name, married Caroline Scott, an Unst lass. I never asked him but presume that was why he had come back for a second tour of duty. Most were understandably glad to go back to the Mainland. Some others became deeply involved in some way in Unst, realised gradually the good points in island living and were very sorry to go. At one time so many girls were marrying airmen there was an imbalance in the population. If the local young men wanted a wife they often had to look outwith the island, probably refreshing the gene stock as a result.

I was an affiliated member of the officer's mess at Saxa Vord. To begin with there were no married quarters, in fact a single

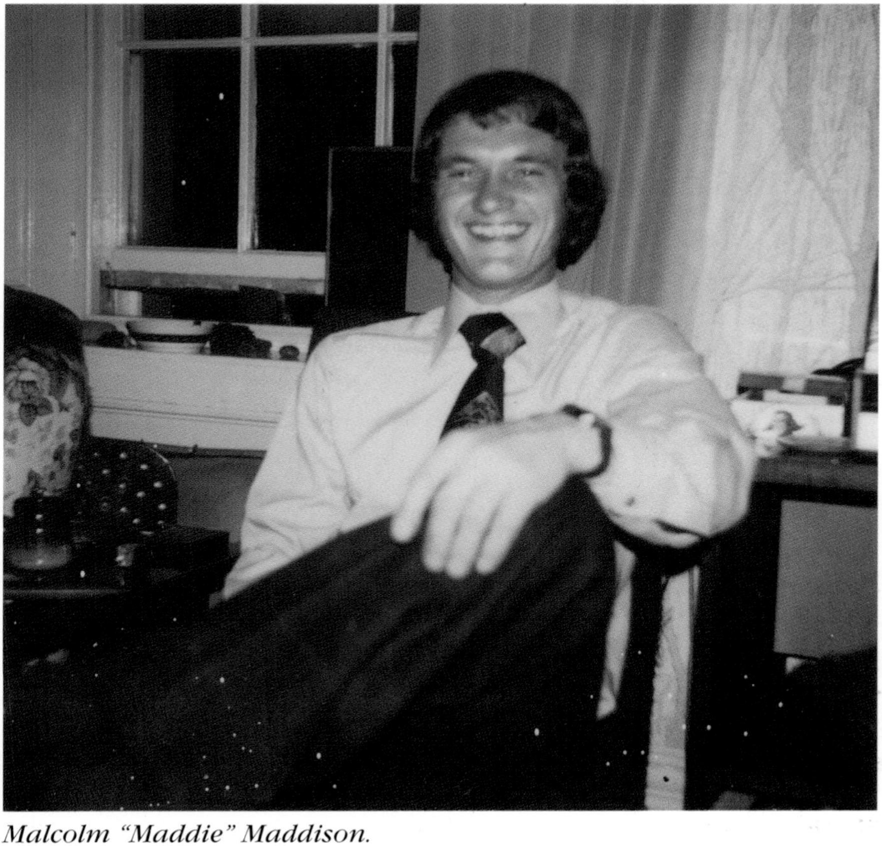

Malcolm "Maddie" Maddison.

posting to all unless they could find a house to rent. As a result any reasonable empty property was hired out. The result was an officer's mess with only a dozen or so officers and few wives to attend social functions. Dining-in nights were strictly male events, ending in horseplay and various games more suited to the junior officers though everybody took part. Unfortunately the dress was formal; my dinner suit wore out fairly quickly and I had to renew it.

Gradually married quarters were built and the mess became a much more sociable centre, especially when the powers that be very sensibly decided to invite ladies to all mess functions. These consisted of dinners about once a month, an odd games night (not involving the rough and tumble of male nights), film shows and, once a year, a dance. Ladies had to be imported from Lerwick for the last event to try and even the numbers. One Lerwick girl met her fate at one of these dances: Lesley Cheyney married a young junior officer, Harry Cairns. He was later to come back as CO.

The officers at Saxa Vord were almost always very sociable and good company. We enjoyed the social events very much, particularly as they were different from the local ones, particularly the chance to be served a nice dinner in very pleasant surroundings, not available anywhere else on the island. Many of these people are still in touch, albeit perhaps only at Christmas.

The Station Commanders also did an eighteen-month tour of duty and they did not interfere with my side of things. Now and then they would need some information or called me in to give me some.

One such incident caused me a certain amount of amusement, though the circumstances were somewhat similar to the scanner situation. The CO left a message at sick quarters with the corporal – would I call along his office next time I was in the camp. I did this on my way out, his office being near the main gate. The CO closed the communication door through to the adjutant's office and proceeded to unlock his safe. He withdrew a document which was for my eyes only. It was almost a 'Robbie' situation.

When I read the papers I could hardly believe my eyes. This was official guidelines for medical officers on how to recognise homosexual officers. All the well known affectations and mannerisms were detailed. I read it with a straight face, handed it back to the CO, who then locked it back in the safe. This was a result of the infamous Burgess and McLean spy scandal. I can report that I never saw any officer holding his teacup with his little finger extended.

VIPs visited now and again. The Air Officer Commanding made an annual inspection which was announced some time previously. The whole camp was titivated up. The old military saying prevailed: 'If it moves, salute it; if it doesn't, paint it.'

On my way up to sick quarters my second-hand Land Rover produced some smoke from the ignition switch when it was started and the same thing happened when I was leaving. I stopped at the MT section and explained the problem to the sergeant there. He agreed to have a look at it, but said it would take half an hour. The wait did not matter when I had the mess to go to. To my surprise all were in their best uniforms, standing round with sherry glasses in hand while the object of attention was obviously an Air Marshall.

"Come and meet the AOA, doctor."

The CO introduced me and I started to chat. "I don't normally come in here at lunch time but there seems to be a problem with the ignition switch on my car so I have left it at the MT section so that they can have a look at it," I said. The CO was making faces at me and shaking his head while I spoke, but I could not understand his signals.

When I spoke to the CO later, he told me the AOA had not long before asked if the MT section was used by any civilian car owners. The CO had vigorously denied any such irregularity. I was obviously so innocent and honest with my story it did not cause any problem for the CO. The AOA knew also that I was the camp medical officer, and anyway he was an extremely nice man who would not have taken the misuse of the MT section very seriously. In a relatively small world, where careers were dependant upon reports by senior officers, I could understand the CO's discomfiture.

As the road reached the top of the hill before descending into Haroldswick, the whole of the sea right down to Balta Isle from Clibberswick would be taken in at a glance. One day my eye caught some movement of ships. Bird watching in a small way had entered my life following the spotting of an avocet near the Westing junction the previous year, requiring binoculars to be carried in the car at all times. I used them to look at these two ships. They were destroyers, steaming in a northerly direction at speed. What was significant, however, was their swept back funnels. Foreign, probably Russian, I thought.

I proceeded to a croft not far from the bottom of the hill to see an old lady who never went beyond the door of the croft house.

"Did you see da waarships in da bay?" she asked, after the consultation was completed.

Yes, I agreed I had seen them and that I thought they were Russian.

"Dat's whit I tocht," she replied.

I proceeded to do the sick parade at the camp and on the way out thought I would ask the CO if these ships were indeed the Cold War enemy. After all, his radar could spot planes from Russia as they came over some distant horizon.

"What ships?" he asked, incredulously.

"Destroyers which looked Russian to me, in Haroldswick," I answered.

He obviously did not know anything about them, telling me to report anything like that if I saw it in the future. I was tempted to give him old Ina Priest's phone number!

One Saturday night about 1am, the phone rang. It was SAC Jones from sick quarters. "I have been called to a man who is very drunk in the billet, his friends are worried about the way he is behaving as a result, what can I do?"

After some questions it appeared the patient was quite conscious but was still drinking. I advised him to take the inebriated one up to sick quarters therefore removing him from further alcohol, to get him to drink a cup of salt water to try and make him vomit, and then to keep an eye on him. If there was any concern to phone me back and I would come up and see him.

I heard no more and found the outcome had been quite satisfactory when I enquired at sick quarters next day. While there, the CO phoned and asked me to look in on my way out of camp. This I did. "All I wanted to do really was to ask you why you called out the fire picket last night?" he said.

I was a bit taken aback as well as mystified. On further enquiry I discovered SAC Jones had called it out, he said on my instructions. They had been sent down to the beach at Norwick to get a bucket of salt water! Fortunately, the CO saw the joke and enjoyed it. Naturally, I had my leg pulled for some time afterwards in the mess.

Following sick parade there was a branch surgery for any local patients. The RAF/local relationships were very good so emergencies in that area were often taken to sick quarters and the orderly there did what he could and informed me. One young girl aged about 10 lived nearby and after being called on three occasions within a short space of time to remove foreign bodies from her nose, I decided I would have to give her a telling off. When I did this I asked her why she repeatedly put things up her nose. She did not answer, but her mother said, "She does it so she can come and see you." I kept a straight face and, hoping my manner was frightening her sufficiently, threatened to send her to the hospital in Lerwick next time she did it. It seemed to have the desired effect as she never did it again.

Chapter 12

Real winter

IN 1960, when I started in Unst, there was only one way of transporting patients in an emergency to the Gilbert Bain Hospital in Lerwick. There was no ambulance in Unst so a mini-bus was utilised instead. The 'ambulance' driver was Graham Hunter who most willingly turned out at any time of the day or night when requested. He completed the first stage of the journey to Belmont.

However, before contacting Graham, it was essential to speak to Davy Johnson in Yell to make sure the weather conditions would allow a crossing of Bluemull Sound. Sometimes a delay was requested until the tidal conditions were more favourable but there was never a situation when the small motor boat did not make it across. Although this service was appreciated by the people in Unst, and none more so than me, I doubt if the dangers were fully appreciated. Davy Johnson and his crewman saved many lives by crossing this very tidal sound on bad winter nights.

Having cleared the Bluemull crossing, the next phone call was to Johnnie Leask in Westsandwick in Yell. At least he ran the Yell Sound boat as well as the mini-bus used there as an ambulance, so the one phone call co-ordinated stages three and four. He then gave me an estimated time of arrival at Toft on the Mainland.

Now Graham was phoned and asked to pick the patient up to be at Belmont at a set time, and lastly the hospital in Lerwick was contacted to arrange for an ambulance to meet the ferry at Toft and to discuss the patient with the surgeon or one of the Lerwick GPs if the patient was medical.

In those days, Ronnie Cumming was the resident surgeon and he would accept any surgical case, however specialised. All the GPs in Shetland were very appreciative of the service Ronnie gave, being entirely on his own for so many years. It was one thing to be always on call for a limited number of patients, and an entirely different one being on call for the entire population of Shetland.

The entire trip from Unst to hospital took from three to three and a half hours at its best, not a pleasant journey for a seriously ill patient. To add more apprehension to the patient, he or she had to be passed out on the stretcher over the stern rail of the

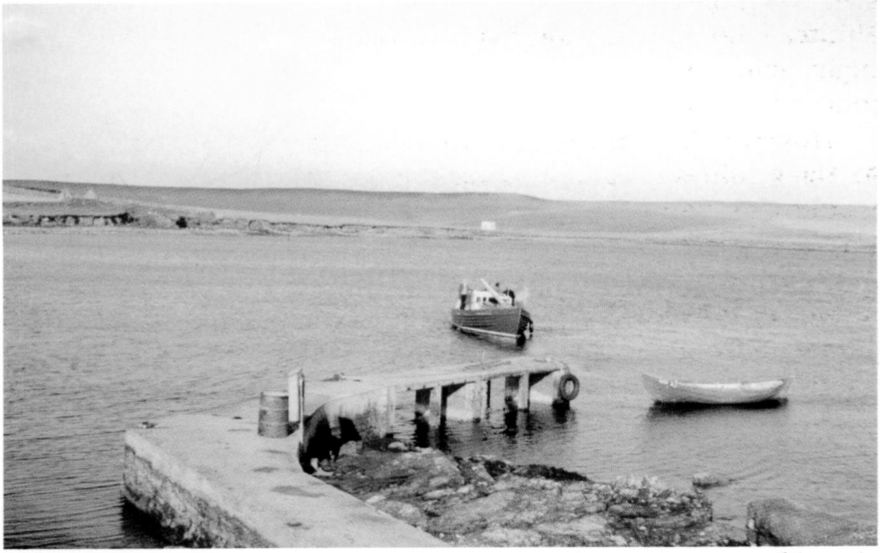

Relief ferry on Bluemull Sound approaching Belmont Pier, 1961.

Tystie to pass down the hatch aft into the cabin. This, of course, had to be repeated in reverse at Gutcher. This proved too hazardous for one very heavy, obese lady I sent off with an acute abdomen. The two crewmen did not have the strength to hold half the stretcher out over the stern rail so she had to make the trip lying on top of the cabin covered by a tarpaulin. It was at least a reasonable night, from the weather point of view.

For the first part of my time in Unst the weather forecast played a big part in life because of these restrictions. An acute appendicitis is sometimes difficult to diagnose, particularly in its earlier stages. However, if the forecast was for a gale imminent, there was no time to wait until the symptoms and signs had fully developed. A balance between waiting and sending in early had to be struck with the policy of 'better safe than sorry' adopted.

It rarely snows with the same regularity today as it did in those years in Unst. Most winters produced a heavy fall of snow, usually with wind so that complete road blockage resulted. This was particularly so in Baltasound along the back road where walls caused the snow to fill in until level with the wall tops. The house and the surgery being at one end of this long straight road, and the antiquated snow-plough which could not clear really heavy drifting, meant even my Land Rover could not go anywhere.

One of these snowfalls accompanied by a very strong wind completely blocked the roads in Baltasound, but the snow was blown off the fields so that each dyke had a long incline of snow both sides of it. I had a patient in Burrafirth on daily injections at that time. I asked for snow plough assistance. The snow plough was a remnant of the Second World War, being a high clearance truck with chains on the back wheels and the typical blade mounted on the front. It lay all year at Spragatup in Haroldswick with the result it was always a surprise the engine started when it was needed. The plough eventually cleared the road to the Kelda junction where the back road in Baltasound started. I was at the other end of the two and a half mile straight. This part of the road always defeated the snow plough and it did on this occasion also. This meant a relatively easy walk across the fields as far as Kelda, carrying my bag of tricks. However, when I came to the walls I found I eventually stepped into snow up to my middle, making it almost impossible to extract my legs or make further progress. I discovered 'swimming' was the answer. I lay down on my front, pushed my bag ahead of me, then paddled up the incline, over the top, then slid down the other side head first. When I reached the corner the snow plough took me to Burrafirth then returned me to the same place for me to repeat the walk and swim back to the house.

Later on I acquired a pair of snow shoes from Canada. They were like tennis racquets strapped to my feet. Unfortunately, they gathered a great weight of snow on top of them each time my feet sank into deep snow so that a sort of wet cat foot manoeuvre was required with each foot as it was lifted. It was like the Hokey Cokey, shaking it all about, but quickly became exhausting so that I gave them up. I borrowed a pair of cross country skis the next winter for a trial period. It was possible to glide well provided there was snow cover but exasperating to have to take the bindings off at each fence or dyke then strap them on again.

One January, just a day after New Year, after a day of snow with a gale, it became heavier as darkness set in. It was going to be impossible to venture out so I did something I rarely ever did and that was to close the Land Rover in the garage. The garage door was never closed normally, a sign of laziness to avoid the difficult task of getting the two halves to revolve on tracks inside the garage on each side.

I had no sooner built up the fire and settled with a book when the phone rang. SAC Smith phoning from Quoys, quarter of a mile off the Burrafirth road, to say his wife was in labour with her first confinement. Instructions were given on what to do if she should deliver without doctor or midwife. Oilskins, rubber boots, extra clothing put on, the garage doors opened after digging, the shovel thrown in the back of the Land Rover with two maternity bags, then two phone calls: the first to John Sutherland at Spragatup, the snow-plough driver, and the second to Carrie Jamieson, the district nurse, health visitor and midwife. It did not matter why or when I phoned Carrie, she was *always* ready to carry out any nursing duty, no more so than that night in blizzard conditions. I told her I would pick her up from her house in ten minutes. She had to get her equipment gathered ready and get properly dressed for the journey.

Three quarters of an hour later I was still digging uselessly a hundred yards from the nurse's house. I could not see for fine snow and my digging efforts were blind but the effort was like peeing in the ocean and expecting the tide to rise: one shovel out resulted in two filling in. I eventually abandoned the effort and

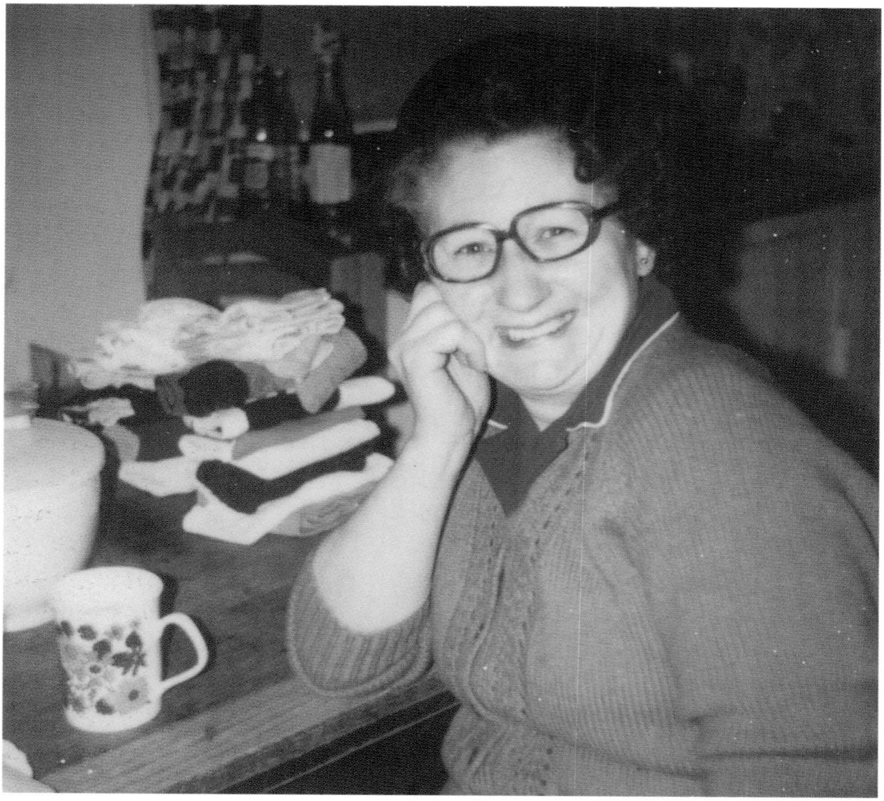

Carrie Jamieson – my right-hand woman.

struggled up to Carrie's to wait for the plough. He eventually appeared an hour and a half later. When I explained my problem he borrowed a rope from a neighbour to pull the Land Rover out. This was eventually achieved, but foolishly the rope was returned to its owner before we set off, Carrie and I following close behind the plough.

Progress was very slow indeed at the Kelda corner, the plough having to reverse then charge each drift in turn. We just had to sit and wait so that by the time the road was clear the Land Rover was snowed in yet again. No rope! John Sutherland had to take down the truck's spare wheel, remove its chain and this was used instead. This meant even more delay and my hands were not very clean by this time. We had just got underway again when the plough stopped. I went out to see what the problem was. John thought he had run out of fuel! The truck was so old it had no fuel gauge. A dip stick in the form of a long starting handle was inserted into the tank and with great relief there was some fuel in it. After a struggle, the engine fired and we started our slow convoy yet again.

When we came to the branch road into Quoys, the Hydro man for Unst, Andrew Laurenson, was waiting there to get into Quoys as there had been a power failure. At this point John Sutherland said he would not go in the branch road as his orders from somewhere higher up were to drop us at the road end. I could not believe this. Poor John was obviously uncomfortable with his instructions. How could the nurse and I carry three or four cases with other bits and pieces for a quarter of a mile on a night like this when the time was now 1am. I had left the house at seven so what was happening in this isolated croft with no electricity and a luckless, untrained husband, probably at his wit's end. I threatened to let all Hell loose if we were left there so the plough did go in the road as far as the croft which lay a hundred yards across a field below the road. Andrew Laurenson jumped off the back of the lorry and disappeared while Carrie and I trudged over the field to a glimmer of light from a candle in the croft window.

We came in just as the head was appearing and I delivered the baby there and then with no time to even sluice my rusty, oily hands. Carrie, meantime, unpacked the essentials as quickly as she could. Everything went fine from there on and by the time we left the electricity was back on.

It was nearly 3am. The plough had gone home, leaving Carrie and myself to make our own way back. Fortunately it had stopped snowing and had become a very cold, frosty night with a strong northerly wind.

We made it up to the Kelda corner without much difficulty and knowing the likely state of the road from there on, I stopped before turning into the back road, telling Carrie to sit still until I explored ahead. As far as I could see there were three huge fans of snow, then less beyond. Going back to the Land Rover I told Carrie to hang on like grim death and gave the vehicle the gun round the corner. We hit the first drift and all went black with snow right up over the windscreen. We hit the second with much reduced momentum and shuddered to a stop. There was no option left to us but to start walking and this we did over the crisp fields to the right of the road.

We plodded on over the next two miles or so until Carrie left me to go down Gutter Street to her house on the left. My mind, like the lost desert wanderer obsessed with water, was likewise full of the great feed of bacon and eggs I was going to make myself when I got home after, of course, a liberal dram. It was 5am by the time I got into the kitchen. I was exhausted, had a glass of water and collapsed into bed.

Follow up over the next few days showed no ill effects of the lack of aseptic technique, but when I suggested the Smiths call the baby boy 'Rusty' I don't think the parents saw the joke.

This was just one of many adventures Carrie and I had together, mainly at confinements, albeit none more adventurous than this one.

Chapter 13

Norwegians

THE economy of Unst at that time depended entirely on the RAF station with a few jobs in the quarries, on the roads, and in service industries. Looking round for some alternative employment which might act as a boost or insurance to what was already in place was not easy. A small development committee was formed to discuss this problem with a view to encouraging another line of employment. I found being a member of this group a challenging and stimulating experience. The local minister, Douglas Lamb, volunteered to act as secretary and off we went.

In Shetland, Whalsay in particular set the pace as far as fishing was concerned, so it was decided that with the fishing grounds being within easy reach of Unst, we should enquire if there was any interest in the island. Having discovered there were some young men keen to go to the fishing the next question was how to resurrect an industry long since dead. Contact with the Highlands & Islands Development Board and with Prophet Smith, who was a member, and Jim Lindsay, their fishery officer, meant many meetings to plead a case.

Eventually a boat was promised and training for the potential crew arranged by personal contact with Whalsay fishermen. It was a proud day to see the *Sapphire* arrive at Baltasound with high hopes she would form the nucleus of more boats later.

About this time the economy of Yell was in a poor way and there was a desire by the Council and the Highland Development Board to try and improve the situation. A Norwegian businessman, Henry Krantz, appeared with a Norwegian crab canner, Sigurd Løkeland, hoping to exploit the untapped crab round Shetland.

A public meeting was held in the Mid Yell Hall to discuss this project, the suggestion being to build a crab cannery in Yell. One or two of us went over from Unst to the meeting. The hall was packed full and the audience very enthusiastic for the project. This was in no small way due to the inspiring address by Henry Krantz who impressed the audience with his sincerity and transparent honesty. I myself was completely won over by him and, as I later got to know him very well, found all my first impressions to have been correct.

Henry had been in Shetland during the war on the Norwegian sub-chasers which replaced the fishing vessels of the 'Shetland Bus' operations. His story is interesting and I will divert a little to tell it.

Henry, at 18, wrote some derogatory remark about Hitler on a wall in Bergen and shortly afterwards found the Gestapo on his trail. He escaped because his older brother Per confessed to the crime. Per was sent to a concentration camp but survived.

Henry was passed along the escape route to a small fishing village north of Bergen to wait with several others for transport across the North Sea. They hid in an old boat house and the only food the local patriots could spare was salt fish and porridge. Later, Henry would eat anything but drew the line at any of the above two items as a result of weeks with nothing else. He eventually came over to Shetland like so many other refugees and was sent to London. He became a petty officer in the Norwegian Navy and was sent back to Lerwick in control of half a dozen Norwegian sailors.

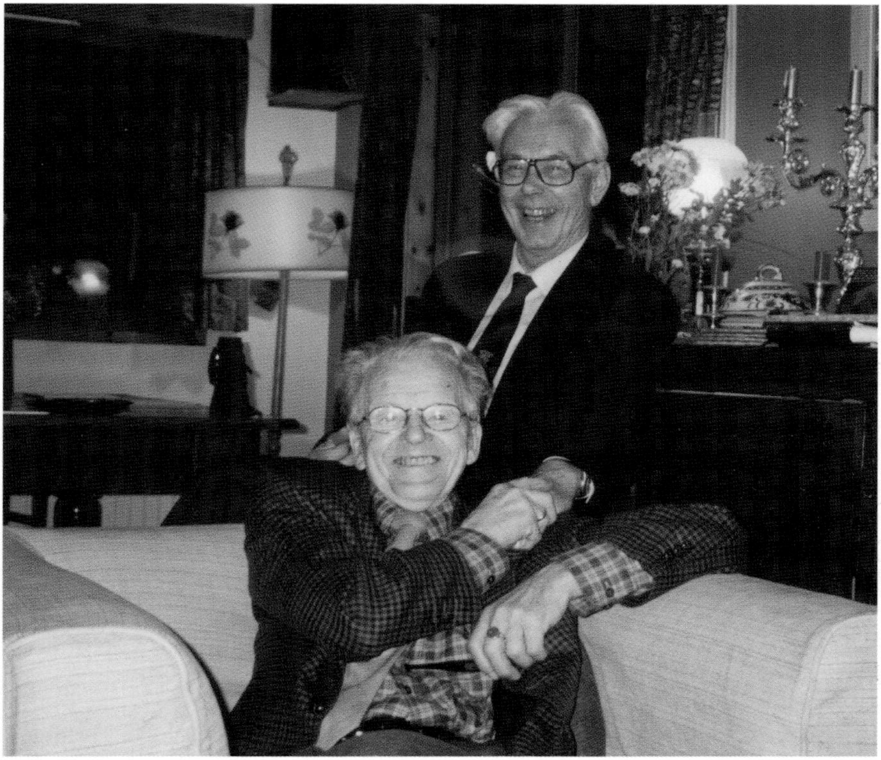

Two very good Norwegian friends of the author: Henry Krantz (bottom) and Edgar Hartvedt.

Before leaving London he was given a ten-shilling note as emergency funds for the group. On arrival at Aberdeen they found the troop ship to Shetland had sailed so they had to stay for a number of days in Aberdeen until the next troop ship went north. Henry's crew soon ran out of money in the pubs in Aberdeen and appealed to him to give them their share of the ten shillings. This Henry did reluctantly. After the war he got a letter from a government office in Oslo asking him where the ten shillings had gone. This involved Henry in a needless amount of correspondence with the Government in Oslo over this trivial amount. Bureaucracy gone mad.

The crab factory which became the Shetland Norse Preserving Company Ltd required added catching power to supply the factory's needs. The HIDB, who had money invested in the factory, now proposed a small fleet of new boats to do just this. Two of these small fishing boats came to Unst, the *Lizanne* and the *Vestra*, helping consolidate a fishing base in the island.

This development committee at a later time formed an action committee to oppose the Zetland County Council Bill when the oil industry started to appear in Shetland. Baltasound was earmarked to become an oil service base, the council having powers of compulsory purchase at valuation. The land most suitable for the service base included all the arable land in Baltasound. There was no proper consultation with the people concerned and what was as bad in many ways was the secrecy and lack of information on the council side, while the private developers visited Unst frequently, were only seeking a small area of land on the south side of the voe for which they were prepared to pay a much more realistic price, and whilst having no illusions about their profit motive went about their business in a much more approachable way. In the end nothing came to Unst, the council being defeated on that part of the Zetland County Council Act. The story of that period is involved and political. It could be dull for anyone not interested so I'll not go into the details.

My acquaintance with Henry Krantz grew mainly because of the lack of accommodation in Yell. He came across to Unst after a day in Mid Yell then travelled back the next day having stayed the night with us.

Shortly after the Shetland Norse factory got into production, Løkeland was bought out and Henry asked me if I would become a director of the factory. The other directors were either in Norway or England so that certain legal documents and, for a time, cheques requiring a director's signature had to be sent to Norway then back again. It made sense to have this facility in Shetland and so I accepted. It has been a long and happy relationship with Henry and his son Pål, the other directors past and present, and also their wives. The meetings were sometimes long and intense but there was always a very enjoyable social evening when that was over. Conversation including jokes in English was no problem to all the Norwegians involved, an ability one can but admire.

The Mid Yell factory is today one of the main sources of employment in Yell so has fulfilled one of its functions. The

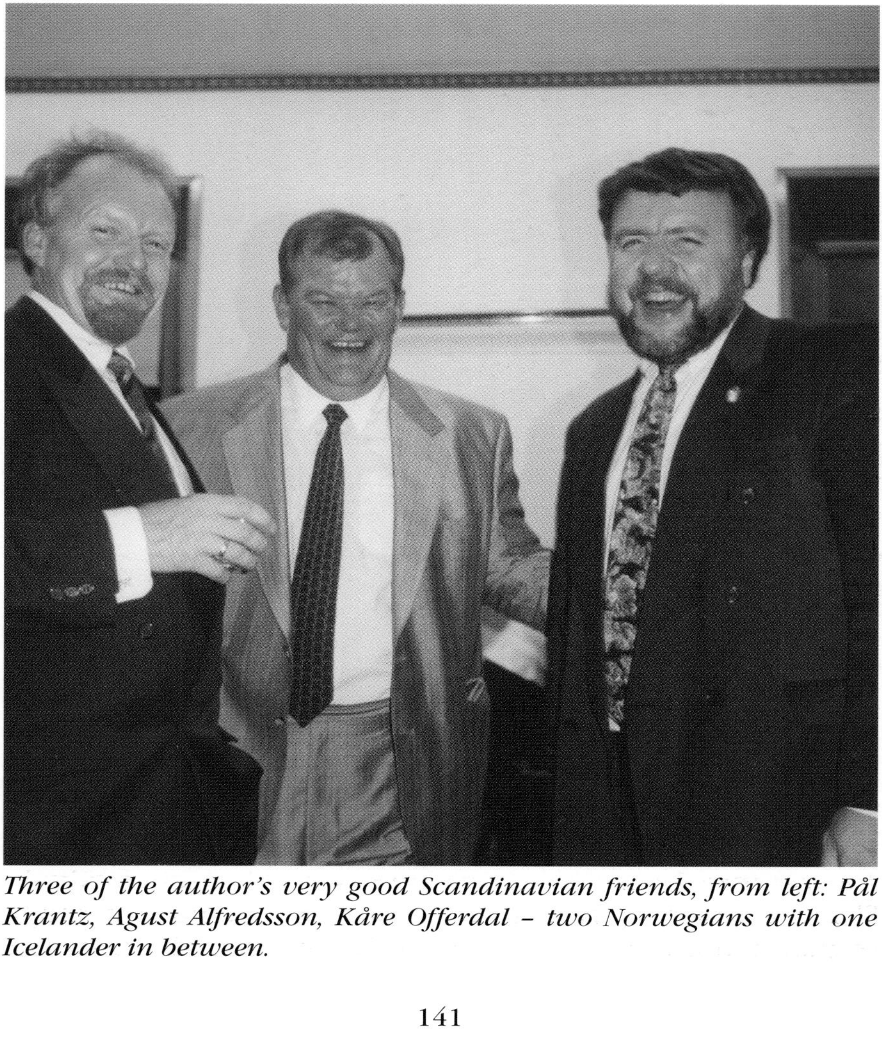

Three of the author's very good Scandinavian friends, from left: Pål Krantz, Agust Alfredsson, Kåre Offerdal – two Norwegians with one Icelander in between.

Shetland Islands Council and Highland Development Board shares were bought back by the company some years ago, allowing the business to be controlled entirely by the directors and shareholders at that time.

Chapter 14

Rules of engagement

A NEW doctor in a rural practice attracts a lot of custom initially. Some come just to see the new incumbent, others to try for the elusive remedy which predecessors have failed to find for them, a few who have stored their complaints because of dissatisfaction, unrealistic or otherwise, at previous visits, the handful of constant attendees, and one or two with immediate needs.

So the surgeries to begin with were very busy. It was easy for the patients as I was the only doctor, but difficult at the start for me because of a number of common surnames. There were also many with the same Christian name, for example there were no less than three John Henry Priests, and three Andrew Stickles. Priest was a common name so that some RAF people were firmly of the opinion it was an entirely Roman Catholic island after finding Priests living here and there. Patients tend to think that if they have seen the doctor once he will remember them and their problems in six months when next they appear. I thought I would never get them sorted out, trying hard not to give myself away but having furiously to identify from the clues they gave me. Little did I think at that stage that by the end of eighteen years not only would I know everyone of them and what their medical history was, but also most of the inter-relationships in the island.

One of these early patients, a male, stated he had come for some medicine for his old mother. I asked him what she suffered from and his answer was headaches. I was just about to explain to him that I could not prescribe for her but would need to examine her when he volunteered the cause of the headaches! "Hit's da new wireless I got dat gees her da sore head. Hit's the atmospherics aff o' it. I want a bottle for dem."

Not being that long out of university and my therapeutics being fresh in my head, though my dispensing limited in choice, I disappeared behind the door of the cupboard which held the drugs, partially to hide my amusement, but also to try and solve this thorny pathology which I had not come across before. Like Spew Campbell, with a self control I didn't know I had, I poured out a bottle of oil of eucalyptus mainly because of its strong medicinal smell, labelled it 'not to be taken' and wrote the directions: one or two drops put in a bowl of hot water placed on top of the radio daily. Next time I was in the house the bowl was in its designated spot and had abolished the headaches completely. This was an early lesson for me in psychological medicine. I suppose the other remedy would have been to keep the radio switched off. Though logical, this would not have been a popular bit of advice and lacked the magic of the bottle.

A doctor in Shetland long before my time was reputed to have a very simple dispensary; he had two buckets: bucket A held a white chalky mixture and bucket B had a brown concoction. No matter what the ailment the patient got either a white bottle or a brown bottle. How he decided I don't know.

It was absolutely imperative that medical confidences remained the secret between patient and doctor. An example, not really an important one except in principle, presented itself one surgery. A lady, whom I knew to be exceptionally curious, followed a seaman off a ship at the pier at Baltasound, into the surgery. The seaman, who was a complete stranger in Unst, had hurt his back lifting off hatches. The lady asked first, "Wha wis yon?"

I did not answer.

"He seemed to be cripple, whit wis wrang wi him?"

Still no answer, but instead a question from me as to what her problem might be. However, she was far more interested in the previous patient than in her own complaint. The question was repeated three times in spite of my efforts to bring her attention to herself. This was more than I could put up with. "Look here, Mrs P., do you want me to discuss your complaint with the next patient when he or she comes in?"

"No, I would not like that."

"Well, that is what you are asking me to do with the patient who has just gone out."

Thereafter we had a perfectly pleasant relationship and she never did it again.

It was also important to me to try and prevent the wool being pulled over my eyes. A new patient appeared at the surgery, a strong, weather-beaten man of about 50, not known to me. He passed the time of day then asked, "Do you like lobster, doctor?"

I fell into the trap by answering in the affirmative.

"I hae a few in the box so I'll bring een o'er fir you."

I thought this was a very kind gesture and offered to pay for it but he indignantly refused. When asked what I could do for him he produced a letter which he passed across to me. This was his undoing for the letter was from the Employment Exchange in Lerwick telling him to appear for work the following week. As soon as I had started to read the letter he said he could not possibly go to this work.

"Why?" I asked.

"I have bad kidneys," he replied, then went on to say he had been in hospital in England with them. I refused a medical certificate until I checked with the hospital and I asked him to bring me a specimen of urine.

I never got the lobster nor the specimen of urine and enquiry revealed no real pathology at the English hospital. I heard later this man refused to turn up for work as he had no oilskins. Apparently lobster fishermen don't need them. He lost his unemployment benefit for two weeks only, then it was restored. I did not have the last laugh but did have the satisfaction of refusing a blatant bribe.

The next day another man came with the same letter but as he produced it from his pocket I recognised it and said I hoped he was not looking for a certificate to get off work. He read the signs immediately and denied it emphatically, stating he had just come for some ointment for his spots.

These two encounters did me a lot of good. Word got round, probably that it was impossible to get blood out of that b..... stone, or perhaps I was called something worse but, anyway, I was never bothered by that type of thing again.

Chapter 15

The sea

THERE was now and again a little more excitement in the practice. I got a call one evening from the RAF asking me to attend a shipwreck at Skaw. I knew the incident was taking place but because we had some folk in the house I could not disappear, much as I longed to do so. A Russian trawler had come ashore at Skaw, in the dark, just inside the Holm of Skaw. The RAF had prepared a hot meal and were standing by to receive the survivors who might need some attention. I excused myself from the company and sped up to Skaw as requested but glad to be in on it. The trawler was hard and fast on the rocks, ten to fifteen feet off the low banks in the area. Lights had been rigged up and the Russians were able, with ropes from the shore, to make it ashore with nothing more than wet feet. Another Russian trawler was lying off in deeper water watching the scene. As soon as the men started coming off, the second trawler launched a rubber inflatable which sped in towards the shore and the survivors were immediately removed and taken off to the ship. It was a quiet night fortunately, my medical services were not required and these men did not get time to be politically contaminated by the people gathered on the shore, at least I presume their rapid evacuation was to prevent this or to stop asylum seekers. There had been the famous Walls incident of asylum seeking previously.

The next day I went up during daylight to see the wreck. Many local men were gathered at low tide but had not made a definite decision to go on board. It was easy to get on board and I made a move in that direction. Within seconds the ship was swarming with men, mostly hauling bundles of herring net out of the hold. A bolder chap removed the ship's bell while I examined the bridge. I found the chart cabinet and removed the charts which proved to be all Baltic. I doubt if they constituted an espionage feat. Later somebody removed the ship's wheel and thereby almost caused a diplomatic incident for a gang of Russians appeared at Willie Sinclair's house at Skaw demanding the wheel back. Apparently it was an airman who had removed it and left it in Willie's barn. Being at the height of the Cold War, any small incident was likely to get out of proportion, so Willie read the signs correctly and handed the wheel over. The

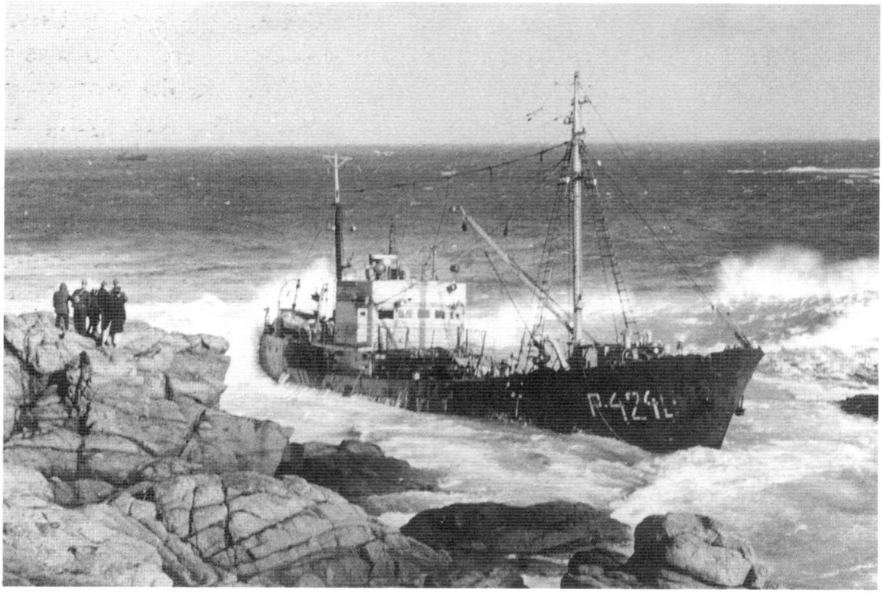

Russian trawler ashore at Skaw.

following day a gale sprang up and within twenty-four hours all that remained of the wreck was a bit of twisted rusty steel poking above the surface.

The phone at Skaw was red hot for a few days with the media making Willie and Charlotte Sinclair's life a misery.

I had a trip in the Muckle Flugga boat to the back of Hermaness one summer day, where a student had fallen over the banks. The only way to reach him was by sea, towing a fourareen to get ashore in. This was a tricky task because of the slight swell but more so because of the slimy condition of the rounded rocks on the shore. Sadly, the unfortunate young man was quite dead. The boat came in again so that four of us could remove the body. It was a grey, misty, damp day when everything is very wet, especially grass. The student had trainers on and he had descended a grassy bank high up the cliffs with catastrophic results.

One very thick foggy Sunday morning about 9am the coastguard phoned me from Lerwick. They had got a message from a French trawler, *Le Matelot*, 60 miles north-west of Unst, asking for urgent medical help. A crewman on board who was a haemophiliac had suffered a head cut and would not stop bleeding. A Peterhead fishing boat, *Ugie Vale*, was lying at Baltasound pier and they were ready to take me to sea to board the Frenchman. This was all very well but a haemophiliac bleeding required refined blood products by intravenous infusion and while I had the transfusion apparatus with some plasma and saline infusion at Saxa Vord, I did not have the necessary fluids. I phoned Lerwick and spoke to Dr Cadenhead but, of course, even the hospital did not stock such specialised products. He agreed to get in touch with the Blood Transfusion Service in Aberdeen in order to get some flown up while I started on the journey by means of the *Ugie Vale*. I phoned Malcolm Maddison at sick quarters to bring all the supplies we had up there to the pier at Baltasound as soon as possible and asked him if he would come off with us. He was the very man I required if I had to set up drips on board.

The fishing boat left at 10am with all our supplies and us two on board. The skipper and crew had given up the chance to have a rest and a sleep by volunteering to go on this mercy mission. They were kindness itself, supplying us with constant mugs of tea and coffee and eventually some lunch when mid-day arrived.

It was as thick as pea soup but with the radio on we could hear a helicopter speaking to the coastguard, the coastguard communication with the trawler, where the language difficulty was causing great problems, then the coastguard asking us for our position. This was after we had been at sea for a couple of hours steering north-west of Balta Isle. The skipper tried to get the French trawler's position but they did not seem to understand so we steamed on.

At this stage I was standing at the starboard corner of the wheelhouse, jammed in between the side of the wheelhouse and the radar because of the oily swell. I was intrigued by a white blip about 180° on the radar which seemed to be coming nearer so I asked the skipper what it was. Nothing of any interest, he said, but I had become hypnotised by the moving spot. Suddenly, out of the fog a mere thirty or forty yards away on our starboard side, a huge German stern trawler came thrashing through the water, rising and falling to each swell. It soon passed us and disappeared in the fog. Nobody in the wheelhouse said anything.

The helicopter could not find us and eventually had to return to Sumburgh for fuel. It had come from Aberdeen with essential blood products and with a doctor on board. A second helicopter then took over from Sumburgh but he could find neither the *Ugie Vale* nor *Le Matelot*.

By three in the afternoon it was obvious we could not find this trawler due to the conditions and lack of proper information of the trawler's position. A decision was made to turn back for Baltasound. In the late afternoon the fog cleared and as we approached Balta Isle there was a stern trawler hove to. It was the missing ship. Maddie and I climbed on board and our many bits of gear were hoisted up after us.

On arrival on the bridge, a fisherman who was sitting there stood up and approached with a bit of bandage round his thumb. This was the patient with a head injury who was bleeding to death. The cut thumb was not even oozing through the dressing. I examined him and he was perfectly fit to be transported on his own feet. This we proceeded to do, lowering all the gear aboard the *Ugie Vale* again. Before I could leave, there was a babble of more excited French and the appearance of another patient. He had a superficial thrombophlebitis in his leg which was not a great problem but finding the appropriate medicine in a large medical cupboard was. This was the first time in 15 years I had had a chance to use my French and I could remember very little of it. I did find what I took to be the tin required and my French stood up to directions before joining Maddie and the patient on the *Ugie Vale*.

The co-operation with the RAF in Unst was such that their ambulance was at the pier. I transferred the thumb and poor Maddie who then had the long trip to Lerwick as escort.

Enquiries later gave equivocal results for haemophilia in the patient. He was flown home the following day.

It was the crew of the *Ugie Vale* I felt sorry for, having used a lot of extra fuel and lost a day's well earned rest for no good reason.

This story does not end there, however. Some years later, John Cluness from Uyeasound phoned and asked me to represent the boat owners at Uyeasound when the Secretary of State visited the following day. He was going to look at the dock at Uyeasound which was tidal and therefore of limited use. I agreed to make their case for improvements when the Minister arrived there.

I turned up at the stated time to find a fishery cruiser anchoring off the pier. The important man, with some officials, came ashore and I did the best I could to convince him of the economic necessity of deeper berths. I then discovered the next part of this official visit was to be to the Shetland Norse factory in Mid Yell. I mentioned I was a director of the factory and so received an invitation to join the party. We went on board the fishery cruiser to be entertained with gins and tonics then a splendid lunch on the way to Mid Yell.

During lunch the Chief Fishery Officer for Scotland asked me to tell the Minister the story of the French trawler. I did so, whereupon he told his private secretary to take a note of the circumstances and he would follow it up when he got back to Edinburgh.

To cut a long story short, I received a letter from the Scottish Office some time later. In it, an apology from the French Embassy in London, but blaming it on language misunderstanding. That Secretary of State was Alec Buchanan-Smith who died quite a young man some years later.

were then fetched to the table and the hostess washed and dried her crockery and utensils before packing everything into a large basket or similar receptacle, which was produced again at midnight for supper and everybody sat down to a feed once more. This meant an efficient clearing away of the tables for the dancing then setting the whole lot up again later for supper. Every third dance, forms were brought out so that everybody could sit down for refreshments. These consisted of whisky, rum, beer, soft drinks and sherry, carried round by groups of willing helpers, including the bridal party. The bridal party remained at the dance until the end.

I always enjoyed the weddings immensely though there was usually a penalty to pay in the way of an after dinner speech. There were so many of these that it was extremely difficult to keep up a new supply of suitable jokes and stories. Eventually I was forced to keep a 'joke file'. Any suitable material I came across was either written down on scraps of paper or cut out of papers and filed in this folder for future use. Eventually I started to write the date of a wedding when something out of the file was used to try and avoid repeating myself. The job was made harder because of the limited audience. Almost certainly some would have been at the last wedding where a particular story was used.

A mild hazard as the evening wore on, particularly in the lobby outside the main hall, was a request for a quick consultation. Only a few tried this, producing readily available areas for inspection. I always tried to be non-committal, eventually suggesting they come up and show it to me one day at the surgery, more than hinting that I was trying to have an evening off.

The 'free' consultation took a funny turn one day when on the way to Belmont to do a call. Just as the Land Rover turned in the Belmont road I got a puncture in one of the front tyres. About 50 yards away some of the local roadmen were standing on the opposite side of the road. In order to get the jack under the front differential in the Land Rover, which was just too far in to reach, you had to be on your back under the vehicle. I had got on my back and was in the process of positioning the jack when I saw one of the men detach himself from his shovel and come across the road. Now I did not need any help, but thought to myself how nice it was for this man to come and offer it. He bent down so that his face was below the front bumper and he could see me under the car then, pointing a finger into his mouth said, "Can you do anything with this tooth doctor?"

I was so let down by this I curtly replied, "Certainly not from this position!" He did not stay, wandering back to lean again on his shovel.

One day, visiting an old lady looked after by her niece, the niece said, "Doctor, I am going to ask you a question I have always wanted to ask you."

I was trying to rapidly recall all the more obscure parts of medicine so that I would not be caught out when she continued, "How do you make oatmeal porridge?"

I was a bit taken aback to think she could not make porridge so I told her, porridge being one of the only two culinary skills I possessed.

One Christmas I was paying a routine visit to an old bachelor who lived alone. "You will have a Christmas dram from me doctor." It was half a question, half an order and knowing how easily he could be upset I accepted his offer. He had many cats so that in the poor light of the croft there was constant movement in the shadows. The first thing he did was to shoo away two cats which were sitting on a dish towel on the dresser. He then picked up the same dish towel to rub inside and outside the small glass. He poured some whisky in the glass and handed it to me, asking if I would like a little water in it. I replied in the affirmative, so he picked up a small jug and went through the door into the byre. Coming back with the jug he poured some water in my glass. I was now waiting for him to stop speaking so that I could toast him with a Happy Christmas. He was standing right in front of me as I sat on the resting chair holding the glass in readiness and waiting for a gap in his monologue, when I noticed a thread-like white object swimming in my glass. At least I had time to consider my dilemma. If I pointed out the wormy thing he would have been very offended and deeply hurt that I had been offered such a thing in his house, but with his whole attention on me, and no flower pot or other receptacle at hand where I could get rid of it, I would have to drink his health. Eventually he stopped, so I wished him the compliments of the season and downed it in one. I always considered this was devotion to duty especially as I am a bit fussy about my food.

About this time I was attending Bertie Neven-Spence at Cocklepoint in Uyeasound. We had become friendly with him and his step-daughter, Marcia Lightfoot. Bertie was a difficult patient for Marcia; he would play up and refuse to take his medicine. Marcia would then phone me and I would have to read the riot act. He was always as good as gold when I had to do this especially as it was an excuse to give me a drink and, of course, have one himself. Bertie had marvellous dreams which he could remember in detail and relate to me if I happened to call. One day he said, "I had a terrible night last night and I am just exhausted today."

I asked why and he proceeded to tell me his dream.

"I was down in Lerwick and as I came to the Market Cross there was a crowd of men trying to manoeuvre the *Earl of Zetland* round the cross and into Commercial Street. I had to give them a hand but she got stuck solid and I am exhausted with all the shoving."

On the road to Uyeasound, about half way, there is a bridge at Watlee reputed to be haunted. There is a story about it in A.T. Cluness' *Told Round the Peat Fire*. This area is remote from habitation so the location lends itself to ghosts, trows, etc. During my time in Unst a ghost car appeared on the main road near there on a number of occasions. I had laughed at the tales until Willie Dodd, the Church of Scotland missionary in Uyeasound, saw it one night. He was a solid Christian man with little imagination so the story of meeting a car in that area, which just disappeared into thin air, began to have a little more credence.

I never thought I would see it myself, but I did. I had got a call to Muness between 1 and 2am, that time when you have to clamber up into consciousness. Still not fully awake as I approached Watlee brig I saw the lights of a car coming from Uyeasound. Being conscious of the Land Rover lights, which are high and close together, I dipped as I came to the brig so as not to dazzle the oncoming car. Another half mile on and there was no car, nor indeed did I meet any car. There is no side road apart from the one down to the Watlee loch and, anyway, that was just after I had dipped for the car which was half to one mile away, so it could not have turned off the main road.

It was certainly a strange phenomenon, probably due to the reflection of lights, but from where? I mentioned it to Brian Hunter years after and Brian, who has both feet on the ground, had had three witnesses in the car with him, one being his wife Margaret. Courage being bolstered by numbers, he had actually gone down the Watlee loch road to make sure it was not a prank, but found nothing.

The only other brush with the supernatural I had was during the day in the company of Maureen, and Nicholas Barnham. We were in Gloup in Yell and decided to peer through the windows of the empty Haa. The kitchen window was not locked so we went in, with no criminal intent, merely curiosity.

Firstly, the clock in this deserted house kitchen was ticking, which seemed strange. Whether it had the correct time or not I can't recall. Then, while in the kitchen, a door closed upstairs and a heavy foot descended the stairs. Now we are in trouble we thought because we have no right to be in here. However, nobody appeared in the kitchen and, after a few minutes silence, we went out into the lobby. Right enough, there was a central steep stair right opposite the front door. However, the door was locked and had a steel bar across it so no-one could have left the house through it. Being three in number leant us courage to go upstairs, to find nothing. I quite recently told Sir Joseph Watson-Cheyne, the present occupant, this story and his wife admits to a female presence which she has seen in the house.

Chapter 19

Evening classes

IT IS a gradual transition from town boy to country boy as I discovered while in Unst. If somebody had suggested before I went there that I might become interested in birds I would have laughed at them. This all changed by a chance sighting of a bird even I realised was different, for its beak curved the wrong way and it seemed to have much more white on it than any bird I had seen before. At this stage I did not carry binoculars in the car but seeing this avocet near the Westing junction, and having it confirmed by someone who knew, changed that.

Of course, the walled garden at the back of Hillsgarth with small trees and shrubs in it proved to be very attractive for birds, especially at migration times. Great excitement to spot a long-eared owl, a shrike, goldcrest, crossbills, waxwings, to name just a few completely new birds for us.

Coming from Hamar one day something strange flew in front of the Land Rover. I stopped and, now having binoculars, saw a great spotted woodpecker attached to the nearest 'tree' (a telegraph pole). Later on we would go anywhere if a strange bird was spotted. My impression was that Unst produced many more species than I ever saw on the Mainland.

What really opened by eyes to my surroundings was something different. It was painting. I had never really known there was a sky there before I started painting. It all came about through a chance remark to my wife that I had always had a desire to try oil paints. I did not know anything about them nor had I even seen them used. At Christmas that year a parcel containing a palette, brushes and oil paints appeared. I secreted myself away and dabbled with what I thought quite good results, so was persuaded the next winter, much against my will, to enrol in the art evening class at the Baltasound school.

That first night at the evening class was almost my last. To my horror, Nick had persuaded a young pupil, Valerie Ball, to sit for a portrait and, to make things worse, Nick handed me a piece of green paper, a stick of charcoal and a piece of white chalk, none of which I had any experience of. However, it is amazing what you can do in a tight spot and the portrait was quite successful so that I have it framed in the house to the present day.

After the initial apprehension, I found this group very good company and their ability more or less matched mine so I went back each Thursday evening with relish. I landed on my feet, however, in having as the teacher Nicholas Barnham. Nick could get results out of any novice painter

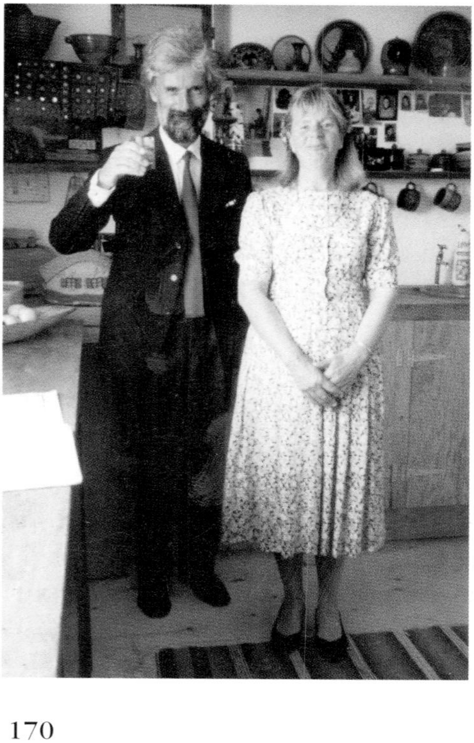

Nick Barnham and his wife Bibi at Mid Ayre, Uyeasound, before a wedding.

and this was nowhere more apparent than in the art produced by the schoolchildren at that time. Not only did I learn a lot from Nick, but came to value him as a very good friend who has introduced me to a wonderful hobby and opened my eyes to the beauty of Shetland.

Another evening class, which lasted only one winter, was music appreciation, run by a teacher who came all the way to Unst one evening a week. He played the piano so that it sounded like a complete orchestra and had that great gift of transferring his enthusiasm to his audience. This did not start my appreciation of good music, but it certainly helped.

To complete my education in Unst I went to the Norwegian class run by Alex Thomson. Alex was a good teacher who made it so much more interesting by pointing out the Shetland word which corresponded with the Norwegian. Place names in particular suddenly began to mean something.

So with such kind and considerate patients whom I was getting to know better and better, with an excellent nursing colleague in Carrie Jamieson, an excellent social life, and all the attributes of an interesting island, I was in no hurry to change it for another practice.

The Executive Council (and the Health Board following them) had a step ladder policy for GPs. This meant that practice vacancies in Shetland were advertised to GPs within the islands before being offered outside. There was an unwritten rule that a practitioner in an island be offered a Mainland post if available. The average length of stay in an island was about five years. When practices on the Mainland cropped up they were offered round. Walls, Scalloway, Whalsay, Yell, Hillswick, Bixter and Lerwick all turned up and each time I declined the offer.

Not long after I started in Unst, Lerwick had a vacancy. I phoned Peter Peterson and asked his advice. "Many a day splatching up a lane in Lerwick getting my feet wet I wish I was back in the country wearing my rubber boots," was his answer. That persuaded me to remain a country general practitioner and I have never regretted it. The Lerwick opportunity cropped up much later again. This time I had been so long in Unst I had first chance. George Smith, my good friend and colleague in Yell, was interested so I had to make up my mind. He took the job when I refused it, then left Lerwick to go to Canada after a few years. When I heard the type of practice George was involved in I knew I had made the correct decision.

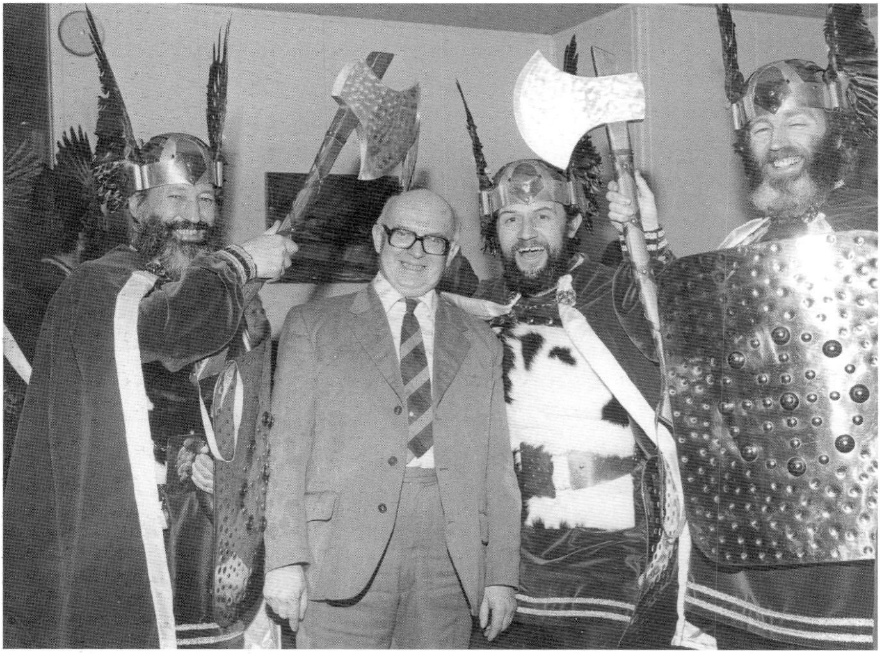

Three Viking doctors and a surgeon at Gilbert Bain Hospital, Lerwick Up-Helly-A' 1977. From left: the author, Ronnie Cumming, George Smith, Ramsay Napier.

Chapter 20

More socialising

I RESISTED the Uyeasound Up-Helly-A' for quite a few years then, on being invited to join a squad one year, agreed to go out with them. The costume was to be skeletons, composed of black clothes with white cloth sown on in the shape of bones. It took a lot of sewing, not one of my strong points, but eventually the big night arrived. The procession finished, we went to the hall which was packed to capacity. No sooner had we got there when somebody touched me on the shoulder and said I was wanted on the phone. There was a call to a sick child in Haroldswick. There was no way I could confront a sick child as a skeleton so had to go home and change. By the time I had finished, the idea of getting dressed in this macabre suit and going back to Uyeasound had evaporated.

Whether it was that year or another I am not sure, but it was at Uyeasound Up-Helly-A' that a local hirer lost his bus! Unst had only about 18 miles of road, not including side roads, between Muness in the south-east corner and Burrafirth in the north-west corner so it seemed an unlikely vehicle to vanish. The story as I heard it started at Uyeasound where the nice Shetland policeman from Yell advised the hirer to take his bus home without passengers as he had had a couple of drams. He very wisely decided to take the policeman's advice and set off north forthwith. About two hours later he appeared at another hirer's house in Baltasound and asked for a taxi to take him home, this request being over another dram, the second hirer being in bed at the time. However, before the second character could get up and get dressed the door opened yet again and in came his son and another man from Baltasound. So the scene is now a bedroom one with five characters, the fifth being the second hirer's wife. It is almost like a Shakespearean play where the instructions state "enter two men into the bedchamber". Son's car had gone off the road and the fifth player had given him a lift home. The original hirer now got his lift home. The next day there was a lot of activity in all the side roads in Unst and eventually the lost bus was found intact in a little used track which petered out at the base of Valleyfield and all ended happily thereafter.

Willie Tammie delivered our milk in the first few years we were in Unst. He ran a Land Rover as a taxi after the milk delivery. Going down a steep hill towards Belmont his passengers were astonished when they were overtaken by a wheel going faster than they were. I presume they had developed a severe and noisy list by that time. Willie Tammie always came in on Christmas morning and New Year's morning with 'brown milk' in a half bottle. There was no refusal and I usually had to get out of bed about 9am to participate in this morning cup.

About Christmas time it was difficult to avoid the Christmas dram. It was often brought in a little glass with the whisky running on to the tray which also contained a plate with biscuit and cake. It was almost impossible to lift the glass without spilling more whisky over oneself as well as allowing no room for dilution with water or similar. When I suggested they should not fill the glass so full I was told quite firmly it had to be like that not to lose the luck.

One old lady who lived with her brother always took me through to her bedroom for the consultation. When it was finished she would say, "Would you lik a peerie corn o' something in your mouth doctor?" She would then 'trivel' underneath her pillow and produce a brown paper bag from which she drew a half bottle of whisky. It always had an unknown label and always tasted particularly good. Refusal was not accepted and when I tried to avoid it by false explanation that the next house I had to visit was teetotal, so I did not want them to smell whisky, she consoled me with, "It will never come from this house where you got it." I never did understand her reasoning. It was really a way of saying thank you. Even though I did not want it, I did not have the courage to appear ungrateful.

I attended a number of refresher courses, some worthwhile and others merely useful. While in Unst I applied for a more unusual refresher course at St Edmund's Hall, one of the Oxford Colleges. This took place during the university summer vacation. The course was a two-week one but with a break of a week in between which I spent in London. The lecturer was excellent and the course well structured. The first week was on neurology, that section of anatomy which tended to become a little blurred

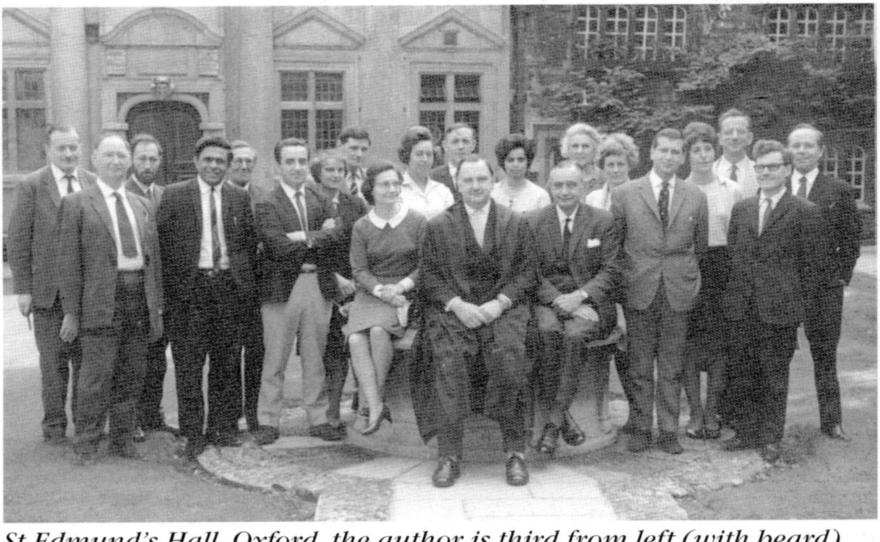

St Edmund's Hall, Oxford. the author is third from left (with beard).

with the passage of time. However, renewed knowledge of the cranial nerves in particular, never goes amiss, as I will relate later. The second week was even more interesting as it was on psychiatry which had not been very well taught at Aberdeen. This course gave me a much better understanding of this speciality and also stood me in good stead when back in practice.

Having finished my course on a Friday, I had to spend yet another night in London before catching a plane to Aberdeen and then to Shetland the following morning. The weather was bad, with a half gale and sheets of rain, but I arrived back at Sumburgh as arranged. I then had to hire a taxi to take me to Toft, followed by a special hire of the Yell Sound ferry when it was a small motor boat. There followed another taxi hire through Yell and a special hire of Davy Johnson across Bluemull Sound. Maureen met me at Belmont and waited until I got home and had some essential food before she mentioned that there was a call to a house half a mile off the road at Uyeasound.

When I arrived there, in my best oilskins I may say, I was ushered upstairs to see the lady of the house who was laid low in bed with severe headache. When I examined her I was astounded to find she had a pituitary tumour pressing on the optic chiasma. My locum, who was a medical registrar in hospital, had not diagnosed the problem and I would probably have missed it if I had not had all my neurology renewed so recently.

I sent her to the neurological unit in Aberdeen Royal Infirmiry and she was operated on soon after. She survived, but died a few months later.

Chapter 21

Obstetrics

MATERNITY patients, if they were to be delivered in Lerwick, had to leave home two weeks before and lodge with friends or relatives in Lerwick until labour commenced. If the expected date of confinement ran over this meant being away from home for up to four weeks which was not only inconvenient but difficult in the case of mothers who already had young children at home. Due to these factors there was an in-built resistance to being confined in Lerwick and in fact, Carrie and I delivered 40 over a period of some years.

I welcomed the chance to practice obstetrics with mixed emotions. On the one hand I was reasonably confident in this field, but well aware of the hazards so that some confinements were stressful but rewarding. Much later I decided I had run the gauntlet successfully long enough and that sooner or later there would be a disaster. Having decided the risks were too great, the attempt to have all deliveries henceforth in Lerwick was not too popular. What then happened was that women nearing term did not go to Lerwick when they were advised to do so but waited until they were in labour and it was too late. I did not mind this 'plunky' they played on me, knowing I had given the proper advice so if they ignored it the decision was no longer mine. I could then attend and do my best to achieve a successful outcome. It never occurred to me to put this advice on paper with the patient signing to say they understood and to have this witnessed; I trusted the patients, naive though it may sound these days, and I think they trusted me.

An early confinement took place in Norwick where I was to experience an old custom which I never came across again. After the whole thing was over, and the patient and baby suitably settled, a tray was brought in by a relative with three sugar lumps on it. On each of these a drop or two of lavender essence was dropped then one lump each given to mother, nurse and doctor. It was, I believe, a stimulant for the mother. Nurse and doctor were surely expected to need revival also.

A forceps delivery in a house or small croft bedroom was a different thing from those I had done in the labour ward. The local anaesthetic technique was the same but the low beds meant that instead of standing to use the forceps I had to sit on the floor. Each time I put some pressure on the forceps my bottom slid on the linoleum and I disappeared half under the bed. Eventually a wooden box would be found to stop this unproductive manoeuvre. To sterilise the forceps there was only one way to do it: no house had a pan with a two-foot diameter to immerse the entire instrument so I used to boil the blades then reverse them to boil the handles. It seemed to work for I never had one case of infection in any of the forceps or normal confinements.

Stitching up after delivery was again not so easy without theatre type lights. More than once I had to do it sitting on the floor while the midwife held a pocket torch, directing the light over my shoulder.

One confinement early in my time seemed to be taking longer than I had expected. I had been hanging round the phone waiting for a call at the second stage of labour. This was the normal routine. Uneasy, I decided to go and see what was happening. The patient was just delivering the head as I came into the bedroom. The nurse had been called away, leaving a relative with the patient. When the baby was born there was only one pair of artery forceps in the dish. Calling in the relative I asked for domestic scissors and found a pair of artery forceps in my pocket. At that time I smoked a pipe so the pocket was always a bit grimy. I washed the two instruments in the sink, immersed them for a minute in some Dettol, then cut and clamped the cord. The baby and patient never looked back.

Another confinement, at 4am (most seemed to prefer the middle of the night), left me with a retained placenta. This was no problem where anaesthetics were available but in Unst, before the air ambulance and no proper anaesthetic, I was in a bit of a spot. Because the patient was a sensible no-nonsense girl, I explained the problem and told her I would have to retrieve it. The anaesthetic, apart from making the procedure much more comfortable for the patient, had another function in that it relaxed the abdominal muscles so that one hand could control the top of the uterus, otherwise it just kept going away from the removing hand. The nurse gave Trilene, a mild anaesthetic used in labour, but not sufficient to give relaxation. The patient was so co-operative that I managed relatively easily to remove a very adhesive placenta. That really decided the issue on home confinements for me.

I never realised that I was getting older until a baby I had delivered, now a young man, got married.

There was one tragedy soon after I started in Unst, due to complete mismanagement by a doctor in Wales. Two young school teachers had moved to Haroldswick, the wife being well pregnant. She came for antenatal care before a holiday period cropped up and they went south for the break. She had some bleeding and went to see a doctor in Wales to see if she should travel back to Unst. She should have been admitted to the nearest obstetric consultant's unit there and then, the faster the better. Instead, she was reassured and set off on the long, difficult journey back. They arrived in Haroldswick in the early evening and at 1am I got a call from the husband to say his wife was bleeding a lot. I knew these people and when he said a lot I could not get there fast enough. The situation which met me was calamitous. I got a drip of plasma going but I only had one bottle so sent saline to keep the intravenous line open at least until she reached Lerwick. The old overland route was set in motion and within three-quarters of an hour she was on her way with the nurse and husband in attendance.

In spite of heroic measures in the Gilbert Bain, including a caesarean section when the patient was not really fit for it, she later died. There is a condition where bleeding does not stop in spite of transfusion and it was this which the poor girl succumbed to.

Chapter 22

Unusual patients

AS I have said earlier, I had a close acquaintance of my headmaster, A.T. Cluness, when at school. By the time I came to Unst he had retired. When I was asked by his wife to come and see him I was very apprehensive. Here was I, a very junior doctor, having to treat the God-like figure of my ex-headmaster who knew only my 'musical skills'!

A.T. was a very wise man of great charm. When I came in he stood up with his hand out and set the tone of the meeting in a few words. "Welcome to Unst, doctor. I am very pleased to see you and to be your patient."

Note how he neatly reversed the situation so that I was the boss and he a mere patient. We got on very well from there on and later he invited me down to this house to play bridge. He was a great bridge player and I discovered how much I was out of his league when, a few weeks after playing, on visiting him, he asked, "Doctor, do you remember that hand where you led the five of diamonds? I have been thinking about it and if you had led the ten you probably would have made your contract."

I could barely remember the evening let alone the hand.

I was astonished one evening later, playing with some other elderly men, on the looks they all gave me on trying to bid a slam.

"We don't play slams," they said, after an uncomfortable minute or so, leaving me with no option but to play four spades and get six. We played on a hoop across our knees which supported a tight cured animal skin, presumably a sheep. With a good peat fire and by the light of a soothing, hissing Tilley lamp; supper was cold mutton, bannocks and tea. Alas that has all gone forever.

On our second Christmas in Unst we invited three of the officers from Saxa Vord down for dinner. There were no wives at that time so otherwise they would have been sitting alone in the mess. We had just finished our first course when a car drew up and in came Jim Hunter, Bertie Henderson and Gibsie Thomson. It was a slightly delicate situation for a moment or two as the two different societies met. I was very glad to see the three of them and did not want them to feel they were intruding but at the same time did not want my guests to feel uncomfortable.

They sat down and I gave them a dram. The conversation was a bit stilted on both sides. Maureen went out to put the turkey somewhere to keep hot while we fiddled with a glass of wine. Then one got up and came across with his whisky bottle. I decided the small liqueur glasses on the table would be big enough so we all had a small dram; then the second; and eventually the third fill of the liqueur glasses. After an hour the whole group was as one and the conversation was non-stop. When they left and the turkey arrived we all had an increased appetite. I think we all agreed it was the best Christmas dinner we had ever had.

Every New Year we looked forward to three first-footers who never failed to turn up. They were splendid company always and many a laugh did we have together. They were Laurie Smith and John and Albert Gray. Albert in particular had a great sense of humour at any time and was always in even better form on New Year's morning. We missed them greatly after leaving Unst; New Year was never the same again.

A new type of medicine would be requested of me every now and again. This was for the perfect patient who did not speak back and where all that was required of me was to do my best with no repercussions if the patient died. I refer to veterinary medicine.

I had no training in this field but with the vet being so far away, my 'better-than-nothing' skills were sometimes requested. All I could do was apply human principles and hope animals were similar to my proper patients. Eventually I purchased a *Black's Veterinary Dictionary* so that I could at least know the normal body temperature of a dog, cat or elephant, though fortunately the last of these was rare indeed in Unst. It was mainly dogs and, rarely, cows which cropped up. The isolation meant a long delay in getting medicine from the vet in Lerwick. As a result I stocked veterinary penicillin. If the vet prescribed it over the phone they phoned me and I sold it to them at cost.

I attended a dachshund which had gone through a window and required a lot of stitching. That paid off in the form of a large sable brush which I still paint with. It was many years later that I discovered how much a large sable cost.

A calf with a large laceration of its nose, having pushed it through a window, also required stitching - not an easy task to try and inject some local anaesthetic into, let alone stitch. A bag of tatties was the reward for that effort.

Two dogs with broken legs, both compound fractures, healed remarkably well. One in particular, a good sheep dog, went on to give many years of good service to its master. They won me a bottle of Drambuie and a bottle of whisky.

We had a cat which was savaged by an Alsatian. There was awful grief among the children so I decided a very large dose of morphia would send it to the cats' heaven. I administered the drug and went back to finish off the morning surgery. When I came out again expecting to have to dig a hole, the cat was jumping on top of the peat stack. At a later date I found out from the vet that morphia acts as a stimulant in cats, contrary to its sedative power in dogs. The cat went on to live its normal span.

We acquired our second Staffordshire bull terrier about this time. He was coming from Aberdeenshire so when old enough we had to organise his carriage. We did not want the pup to be separated from his mother and then spend a night on the steamer. It suddenly occurred to me that the Air Officer in Charge for Strike Command would be flying up in his private aircraft the next week. I put through the CO a polite request which was granted. The pup spent no time in his box in the aircraft, being held on knees and fed by the crew all the way up from Dyce. Loki was the only dog I know who arrived at his future home to be met by a guard of honour.

Chapter 23

Tall stories

THERE were a few 'Robbies' in Unst. They, like grand uncle, told their stories so often they believed them themselves. It was useful, when telling these whoppers, to base them in some foreign place so that the tale had more credence and could not be checked.

One particular man lived in Baltasound but had been in New Zealand. He very seriously told us he had been on a train in that country and had just lit his pipe when an irate lady with a small dog on her lap, having pointed out the no-smoking compartment notice, leant forwards, plucked the pipe out of his mouth and threw it out the window of the moving train. As quick as a flash he reached over and threw the little dog out the window. When the train stopped at the next station who appeared on the platform but the little dog with his pipe in its mouth!

Another character from the south end of the island told a very good story, among many, as incredible as the dog and pipe one. He was at a dance in Uyeasound where a stranger, a pretty girl, attracted the local lads. Our narrator said he would put on a bet that if he asked to see her home she would accept. Right enough, she did. He discovered she was living in such and such a house and when they arrived there she invited him in for a cup of tea. On entering, a man got up from a seat near the fire. The girl introduced our storyteller to him, saying, "This is my husband. I bet him before I went to the dance tonight that I would get the best looking man in the hall to see me home."

This same man told of a terrible gale from the south-east which was causing the sea to break across the road in Uyeasound. He had to drive through this and his car boot lid flew open in a particular heavy gust. Shortly after, a big sea broke over the car and he felt a bump. When he got to the east side he got out to close the boot lid and there, lying in the boot, was a huge olick!

It was the people who made life so interesting and rewarding. In the last few years I was in Unst it was thanks to Carrie Jamieson that many problems in the island were discovered through her duties as health visitor. She was very conscientious in all her work and no request, at any hour, was ever refused.

Taking some interest in medical politics meant attending medical meetings in Lerwick. To do this it was necessary to stay overnight in Lerwick. With the car ferries I could be back in the morning but not before the surgery started, so Carrie would deal with repeat prescriptions, blood pressure checks and such like until I got back. Anything she thought it necessary for me to look at she brought back later. Theoretically, this was not allowed by the nursing hierarchy and Carrie would have been reprimanded if they had known. Duty and loyalty came much higher in Carrie's priorities than rules and regulations. I am grateful for all the help Carrie gave me.

As eighteen years at the practice in Unst approached I began to think it would be nice to have some guaranteed time off. That meant a partnership outwith Unst and my thoughts turned to Voe, knowing Albert Hunter was going to retire. The practice was not quite big enough for two but with the construction of the Sullom Voe oil terminal and all its attendant housing at Brae, Mossbank, Voe and Firth, it was going to enlarge to that size in the near future. I knew I would get the first chance of the practice and I had an excellent potential partner lined up in an ex-Yell colleague now in Aberdeenshire, Dawson Clubb. While home on holiday he expressed a desire to come back to Shetland again; all that was needed was a vacancy, but preferably a partnership. It was now or never and so I applied for Voe.

Chapter 24

Voe

I WAS due to take over the Voe practice on a Friday. Dr Albert Hunter would not hear of it. He said it was bad luck to change on a Friday so I stood at the back while he did his last evening surgery at Voe, and at midnight I took over. The following morning (nothing happened during the night, which was fortunate as I was squatting at Olnadale and Albert had gone home to Gott), I did the Saturday morning surgery.

Maureen was in Unst and I had a bed, a table and a chair in the empty house. A number of problems, like damp in the kitchen, had to be attended to and also redecoration. This took three months and only then did we move in properly.

BP had Voe House as a hotel for their visiting people and in 1978 cost was never considered. They kindly offered me dinner any evening and I took advantage of this once or twice a week. The chef was excellent and there never seemed to be any more than one or two men staying. Maureen popped up and down from Unst and always brought prepared dishes with her. I can't really remember but I presume it was bully beef and beans in between.

Albert gave me a lot of information about the practice on that last evening, including who was related to whom. This, of course,

I could not absorb as I did not know the people, but he knew the complete family histories of most of them.

The first thing was to stock take. Alan Hourie from Stout's chemist came out and counted all the tablets etc., then valued the drugs which I then bought off Albert. Eventually Dawson Clubb would take the Unst practice and pay me for the stock in hand. A year later, Dawson was paying for half the drugs at Voe. Fitments like examination couch, steriliser, chairs, desks, cabinets, etc., were valued by Albert and I and agreement reached.

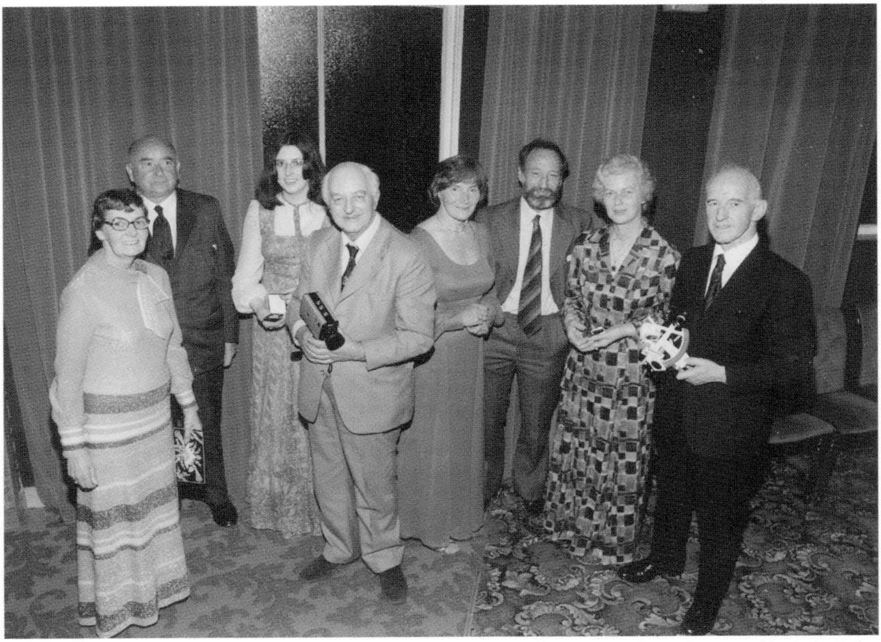

Presentation to Albert and Neil, 1978. From left: Beryl Laing, Peter Peterson, Eleanor Hunter, Albert Hunter, Maureen Robertson, the author, Sheena Cadenhead, Neil Cadenhead.

Chapter 25

Marine operations

WHEN I took over the Voe practice it was in a stage of transition from quiet country practice to a busy, growing one, with industrial medicine becoming part of the job.

Sullom Voe was being constructed, with 4,000 men accommodated at Firth and Toft camps, the excess on the liners *Rangatira* and *Stena Baltica* moored at Sullom Voe.

At the medical centre at Firth, two doctors and fifteen nurses were employed. The drugs for this set-up were ordered by the Voe practice but were dispensed at Toft and Firth by the BP doctors on Voe practice prescription pads. This involved a lot of work at the end of each month when all these prescriptions had to be sorted and counted. I acquired as receptionist from Albert, Averil Blythe, on whom the administration of the practice fell. Averil, though not a trained nurse, used her common sense to keep it all running smoothly until an extending waistline terminated the job. She was valuable to me for her knowledge about the patients and the practice in those early days.

Although the numbers in the practice grew almost daily, the facilities at Voe did not. The waiting room held six people packed in closely, the rest having to stand in the corridor or outside. The surgery was a reasonable size with a very small dispensary off it.

The practice boundary was extensive, from Nibon and Sullom in the north to Girlsta in the south and from Lunnaness in the east to Gonfirth, Stromfirth and some houses in Weisdale to the west. A few patients who moved out of the practice area but who passed our test were allowed to remain with the practice so there were also a handful in Ollaberry, two in Trondra, six in Scalloway, a half dozen in Weisdale, two at Whiteness and even two at Quarff. Home visits to any of these patients took at least an hour or more but they understood the situation so that they never once abused the arrangement and only occasionally a call to the 'wrong' place took more time than was available between surgeries or even after them. The local patients were also excellent and most of the incomers the same.

After a year Dawson Clubb, who had stepped into my empty seat in Unst, came down to join me as a partner. This made a huge difference to the workload though having a single surgery sent one of us out on visits just to get out of the way whilst the other saw the patients at Voe. We fixed up a rota of duty over a fortnight which still existed when I retired. It was a great luxury to plan ahead knowing you were off-call on a certain evening.

Dawson and I had a contract with BP to provide 24-hour cover for the terminal and to do one session of medical examinations up there each week. Sick men on tankers either in the port of Sullom Voe or waiting their turn to come in were attended to via the various tanker agents. This introduced us to added difficulties at times with language. Going on board a Finnish tanker on one occasion meant a medical history being obtained fourth hand; I asked the captain the question in English, he asked the mate in Swedish then the mate asked the sick man in Finnish. The answer was then sent through the reverse process to end up in English again. The sick man spoke only Finnish, the mate Finnish and Swedish, the captain Swedish and English and the doctor only English!

Two men off a British tanker asked to see a doctor. One was an officer from the ship and the other a Chinese crew member.

The crew member was seen first. He came in and announced, "Me go Hong Kong."

I considered that decision a bit premature and insisted on examining his arm or leg or whatever before making any transportation arrangements. I could find nothing wrong with him and said, "You go ship."

"No, no, me go Hong Kong," he insisted.

I was just as determined not to be taken for a ride and terminated the interview by repeating, "No go Hong Kong, go ship."

The officer was then seen with a completely genuine complaint. I told him the Chinese crewman was most insistent on going home to Hong Kong and I had refused. The officer replied in a most apologetic manner, "As a matter of fact that man is useless on board the ship and the captain wants rid of him."

That altered everything. No medical decision was now required from me so I went out to the waiting room and said, "You go Hong Kong."

I went on board a tanker as it tied up one night just after midnight, to see three crew members. When I arrived at the sick berth there were ten others waiting in the corridor. They were Indian and none had any real ailment. They were dismissed with vitamin tablets but even so it was two in the morning by the time I got clear. By way of apology, the captain handed me a bottle of whisky as I left.

I was completely beaten with one Indian crew member some months later who spoke no English but just pointed a finger into his mouth then removed it. I examined his mouth, his teeth, his throat, and could not see anything wrong. It was the most unsatisfactory consultation I ever had, sending him off with an antibiotic in the hope it might do some good.

Peptic ulcers in crewmen sailing from Sullom Voe destined for the States always caused some worry to us. Anything might happen in mid-Atlantic with no possibility of medical help.

At least this part of the practice was different and I always enjoyed going on board ships. A Yugoslav ship doing some survey work in Yell Sound asked for a visit from a doctor on New Year's night. The pilot boat at Sullom Voe took me off and had to wait quite a long time to take me ashore again. The captain and crew were isolated and obviously desperate for company so when I had seen the genuine patient I was seated at a table with candles, given coffee and a newly baked confection of some sort made specially to entertain me. I was then given a detailed tour of the ship and a pound of coffee beans, two hundred cigarettes and a bottle of whisky to take home. I hope I did a little to relieve their monotony in return.

On two summer evenings I had little excursions to tankers: the first all the way to Colgrave Sound, between Yell and Fetlar, by pilot boat, accompanied by the police to a sudden death; the second by helicopter to a Korean tanker lying north of the Ramna Stacks to see an engineer who had hurt his back. This man I evacuated by coastguard helicopter so spent the waiting time drinking coffee on the bridge enjoying the beautiful evening. The Ports & Harbours helicopter then lifted me off and I had the interesting experience of flying over the Ramna Stacks, Fethaland and North Roe back to Sullom Voe, areas I knew quite well from the sea but never before seen from that angle.

It occurred to me that the easiest way to get to the continent from here was by sea on a tanker. Almost every day a tanker sailed to a European destination. Negotiation via John Anderson at Hay & Co., the agents for most of the tankers, produced permission to sail on the German tanker *Friesland* bound for Wilhelmshavn. Maureen and I went on board at Sullom Voe, being allocated the owner's suite. We had full run of the ship, the first mate being delegated to look after us. He did this so well we became friendly and he would appear now and again when the *Friesland* came back to Sullom Voe. The food was good but rather strange, especially to be given egg tartare at 7am for breakfast one morning. I spent most of my time on the bridge, especially when we ran into fog in the German Bight. This delayed the ship considerably so the voyage took two and a half days. Whilst on board we discovered this tanker was owned entirely by doctors and dentists in Hamburg.

Another part of the job at Voe, and later at Brae, was unpleasant and almost always meant work in the early hours of the morning at weekends. This was taking blood at the police station from drivers. At least it was more impersonal than the previous method of deciding on fitness to drive, which meant an examination and then a medical opinion. It was even more difficult when a request to be examined by his own doctor came from the driver. My experience of that was the patient expected a not guilty verdict however unfit they were, and an honest decision sometimes met with abuse.

The Board of Trade and Department of Transport required a doctor to examine seamen and I was approached. New regulations for fitness to go to sea had appeared and this included people like ferry boat skippers and engineers so it entailed quite a lot of medicals but had the advantage of getting to know the people. I have to confess to bending the rules a little now and then for ferry crew in particular. Tug skippers and engineers added to the list requiring medical examination as did all the harbour pilots in Shetland and at that time there were over twenty pilots, probably about twenty-five if I remember correctly.

Having sailed on a tanker from Sullom Voe I felt much more able to decide on the physical fitness required for pilots. Watching the pilot getting off and on to one of the pilot boats in a moderate swell made me appreciate how nimble they had to be. I had also had to climb a rope ladder the night I went to the tanker in Colgrave Sound and I found it a nerve-racking procedure for each time you pulled yourself up with your hands the step seemed to disappear and you had to feel for it with your feet.

Having always been interested in all things maritime I enjoyed this part of the work, finding most seamen down to earth and pleasant to deal with.

Chapter 26

Brae

THE area of the practice being large, there were several nurses employed on the district. One of these looked after Nesting and the south end of the practice. This was Rose Moynes, who had a broad Irish accent. She came into the surgery one day of a flying gale and told us her car had just been missed by a "great big blackboard" in the Kames. We could not fathom out where this blackboard came from until she asked what kind of a "board" it could be. Amidst much laughter we suggested a crow or a raven.

About this time Dr Mike Hunter became a partner with me in a good-sized motor boat. This boat was called *Searcher*. Rose announced one day she had seen our boat at Nesting. We were not very sure if she was right so asked her to describe it. No need, she said, she read the name on the stern.

"What was it?" I asked.

"Sea Archer," she replied, very firmly.

Eventually the Brae Health Centre was built and we moved lock, stock and barrel over there. This gave us two consulting rooms and a dispensary with a small treatment room – at least double our previous accommodation. Averil went off to have her baby and Dawson and I had a great stroke of luck. We discovered

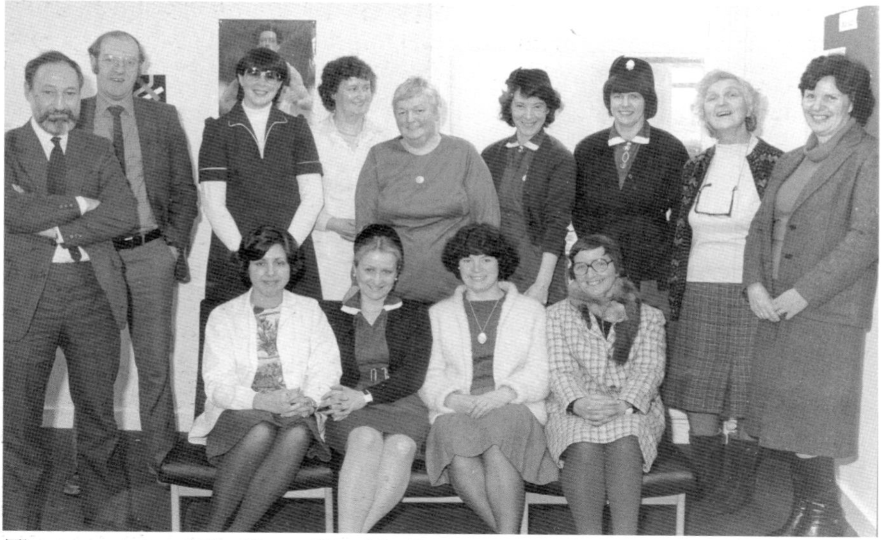

The opening of the Brae Health Centre, 1981. The author and Dawson Clubb with health board employees including Laura Stout (5th left, back), Mary Wood (6th left, back), Nora Peterson (7th left, back), Jill Turner (right, back), Liz Munro (left, front), Rose Moynes (2nd left, front) and others.

a nurse living at Mulla in Voe, married to a BP man, who agreed to come as practice nurse, an arrangement which lasted quite a few years until her husband was posted to Aberdeen. She was Liz Munro, who not only became practice nurse but practice manager too. She reorganised the entire practice at Brae, not only the administration, but Dawson and me as well, in the nicest possible way I may say.

Within a short period of time the workload was far too heavy for one nurse so we took on another, Kay Naisbitt. This formed a happy team again only to be broken up when Kay moved south. What luck we had in finding Caroline Garrick, who became the boss nurse when Liz had to leave, and who was there until recently.

Gradually the numbers of nurses increased until there were four or five, some working part-time, who proved to be great

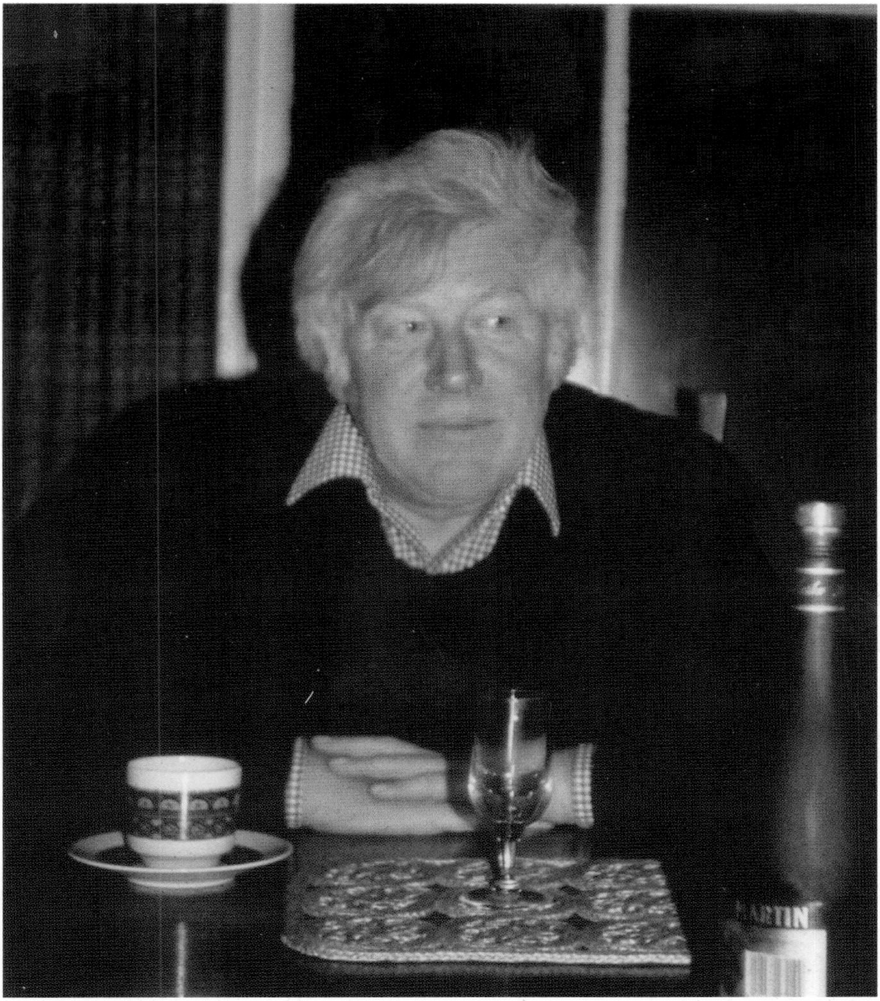

Dr Allan Dowle.

Another of his problem patients complained about the way he was being treated. "We are getting up a petition to complain about you doctor."

"That's fine," replied Allan, "bring it along to me and I'll be the first person to sign it."

Allan had us in fits of laughter when he told us one morning he had said to a patient, "Just jump up on the couch," to find the patient using it as a trampoline.

Northmavine was a favourite painting area and so convenient from Voe or Brae. There was always a break for lunch when painting and on one particular day four or five of us stopped to have a picnic at the Blade of Heylor. We had just started to eat when Lennie Smith appeared, as was his wont. He chattered on without a break, asking a question here and there while we listened and answered between mouthfuls. I was determined not to give him the satisfaction of knowing who we were and managed to avoid the more direct questions. At one stage he volunteered that their doctor was away on holiday and the locum seemed a fine fellow but liked a drink.

"Dir aa the sam, yun doctors," I suggested.

"Yis, yis," he agreed, but followed up with some praise of "Dr Dule, wir ain doctor."

The laugh was on me for a fortnight later I was again at Heylor unloading the rubber dinghy from the trailer to go across to the banks on the other side of the voe. Sure enough, I had barely unloosened one rope from the trailer, when Lennie appeared. "Hello, Dr Robertson," he greeted me. "Man, I kent your grandfather weel; many a time we rowed him up the voe here."

How he found out who I was I never knew.

Those of you who knew Lennie will remember he had few teeth so you had to listen carefully to be able to make out what he said. Having some Norwegian friends staying with us we were 'doing' Shetland and went down to the Blade to see the tirricks nesting there. Immediately, Lennie appeared and we chatted, or rather he chatted, for a while. After he went away Edgar Hartvedt, my Norwegian friend who spoke excellent English and understood it even better, asked, "What nationality was that man?"

He had not understood one word he said.

Mike Hunter told us a good story about Allan. He phoned Mike one day to ask for a bed at Levenwick as he was getting the early morning plane out of Sumburgh the next morning. Mike replied that was no problem and they would have some dinner ready for him when he came down. When he eventually arrived, quite late, he refused the meal, but asked for a large brandy. Mike poured it for him and had a soft drink himself. Allan was a bit indignant because Mike was not joining him with a brandy, even after Mike explained he was on call. However, Allan very quickly asked for a refill. Before going to bed Allan asked Mike if he had an alarm clock and when reassured they all went to bed. At 5am Mike wakened Allan, who complained he had not slept a wink all night. Mike did not tell him that neither Frances nor he had had any sleep because of Allan's snoring in the next door bedroom!

Chapter 27

The good and the bad

LIFE at Brae was hectic and became gradually more so. We extended the surgery times in the mornings by half an hour and both worked flat out to see the patients. By this time we had instituted an appointment system, allowing two patients per quarter of an hour. If the consultation was a quick one we took anybody waiting from our own or the partner's list of appointments unless there was a specific reason for the patient to see one particular doctor. This was a great help when you got bogged down with a complex case or just a garrulous one and were over-running your time. We had a firm rule - any patient wanting an appointment that day had to have one. If we were full up and the patient could wait until the next day, all well and good, but we believed it was wrong to add to further surgeries both from the patients' point of view and our own. Once this starts it snowballs so that there are few vacancies in the appointment book days in advance.

Eventually we had a cup of coffee then started two further surgeries each morning. We kept the afternoons clear, if possible, for routine medical examinations, extra time-consuming consultations, antenatal examinations and minor surgery.

After I retired the doctors in the health centre started afternoon surgeries. The demand appears to be insatiable.

On the other hand, the Shetland patients and the majority of the 'incomers' were extraordinarily undemanding for home visits. As a result, I did fewer home visits than I had done in Unst, for three times the population. The area covered by the practice was so large that if it had not been for such excellent patients I doubt if two doctors could have coped. Apart from Voe and Brae, most calls required at least an hour's time for the furthest out patients.

There were two isolated houses in the practice at that time, now unoccupied, and with a long walk over the hills. The more difficult of the two was Bunnidale on the east coast, half way between Lunning and Leveneap in Vidlin. The family in there at that time had two young children yet it says a lot for the young mother who sometimes phoned for medicine, but never asked for a visit. We admired her self-reliance and application of common sense.

The other isolated patients were at Sandwick, well out Sweening Voe, which I had experience of when doing the locum in Voe earlier. The family consisted of brother and sister and they, likewise, called for a visit on very rare occasions. However, one call which I did, required a form of evacuation I had never used before. In January 1981, the lady of the house had fallen and hurt her leg. She persisted for a day or two but eventually asked for a visit. I went in and could find nothing on examination, eventually putting it down to bruising and perhaps some ligamentous sprain. I left some analgesics with the patient, telling her to let me know if it did not settle in a day or two. Two days later there was a message to say it was no better.

I went in again and imagine my horror to find obvious signs of a fractured neck of femur. Having eaten humble pie the next thing to decide was how to get the patient out. The weather was typical January, almost gale force and heavy rain. The walk out to Sweening was difficult along the cliff edge at the best of times, but with a stretcher almost impossible. I decided to ask the lifeboat to do the evacuation and they very willingly agreed. They had to row ashore in the lifeboat's rubber dinghy, then carry the patient on a stretcher down to the shore and row off to the lifeboat again. They contacted me once the patient was aboard and arranged to transfer her at Toft pier, rather than subject her to the much longer and very rough trip back to Lerwick. I met the lifeboat at Toft and the patient, who was as cheerful as ever, was transported to the ambulance for a much quieter journey to hospital. I am glad to say she did well. We were all grateful to the Lerwick lifeboat crew who did a splendid job in the dark in awful weather.

There were a few characters in the practice who afforded a little light relief now and again. One old fellow came to get his diuretic at the health centre one day. I happened to be the only one available so I dispensed his water tablets and by way of conversation asked him if the tablets agreed with him. "Oh yes," he replied, "I only take them when it rains."

I always enjoyed the late Willie Herculeson, who had the shop at Vidlin. He was full of fun and could keep an absolutely straight face while making the most outrageous statements. One morning in the surgery he asked if he could have some more Clinitest tablets. These were tablets for testing the urine for sugar and were very caustic, so people using them were warned not to get any of the compound on their fingers or, worse still, near the eyes. Agreement to the repeat of these tablets was just a formality and I agreed to write the prescription. While I was doing this he said, "Yon tablets have a hell of a taste." I almost jumped out of my seat and, looking up at him, still took a few seconds to realise he was joking as not a glimmer of a smile appeared. Of course, I was quick to realise, this was Willie at his best.

To enjoy the joke further, I told him to do the same thing to the girls in the dispensary when he was collecting the tablets but to make sure I got into the dispensary first to see their reaction. For half a minute he had them on the hook too but they knew him well and soon realised he was pulling their legs.

Captain Jim Nicolson lived across the road from Olnadale. He was well known to me from school days and had once played a prime role in a leg-pulling operation in Unst. Jim spoke almost entirely in nautical talk, a perfect example being the following: Knock on kitchen door at Olnadale one evening, in comes Jim, "This is a mayday, Bobby!"

"A mayday?" I repeated, not really understanding what he was speaking about.

"Yes," he went on, "June is on a lee shore; she's run out of bunkers."

I was still no wiser until he asked if I had a spare packet of cigarettes!

Jim consulted me at the health centre on one occasion and I suggested I refer him to the visiting consultant from Aberdeen next time he was up in Shetland. His reply was, "That will be fine but I hope he's not one of those who work under a flag of convenience."

I leave you to interpret that remark as you wish.

An older man from Muckle Roe used to collect his prescription on a small motorbike. Clad in windproof jacket and wearing a leather helmet complete with goggles, Liz always referred to him as 'Biggles', a name we always thought was very appropriate.

Unfortunately, not all the patients were interesting characters like the few I have picked out and before long we experienced a different type altogether.

I normally opened up the surgery about 8.30 in the morning to answer the phone before the girls came in at 9 o'clock and to tidy up any paperwork requiring attention on my desk. I opened up the dispensary as usual one morning to find it in a bit of a state. The window was shattered, with glass everywhere, the dangerous drug cupboard had been torn from the wall and the door forced with all the contents gone. I called the police and left everything as it was or as near as I could; by this time the phone was starting to ring and I had to remove the appointment book at least from its place near the window.

It was not easy to have surgeries going on with the CID taking fingerprints, etc., in the midst of the shambles. It was like an ice-house with no window so as soon as the police were finished we got a local joiner to re-glaze the window. The police caught the burglar as they knew who the possible culprits might be and on visiting one he admitted the crime. We even got our dangerous drugs back from their hiding place. I am glad to say the criminal was not from Shetland.

We were to have this happen to us another twice. On both occasions a specific drug was stolen and traced to an incomer living in Brae. To do it once was bad, to break in again and steal the same type of tablet was stupid as the finger pointed directly to the culprit. At a consultation with Dr Clubb shortly after, this patient knew he would be sent to prison but his only worry was which one. He did not know anything about Aberdeen and hoped it would be Barlinnie in Glasgow, where he had lodged before, as he could get any drug he wanted in there!

We had a problem with another incoming patient who would go down to England and get a prescription for a hundred tablets which we refused to prescribe here. We wrote to the doctor concerned but he persisted in doing it on at least a further two occasions. If it had happened again we were going to notify the General Medical Council and complain. We presumed this patient then sold the drug at great profit but may have consumed them personally, we never discovered which.

A constant guard had to be kept for the temporary resident with a convincing story of chronic pain requiring certain analgesics. There were frequent warning notices from the health board about certain people who might turn up. We did come across one. When we refused, he managed to con another GP in Shetland and obtained what he wanted.

However, these unwelcome facets of the practice were as nothing compared with family 'X'.

As the oil industry started to contract, many houses built for the oil boom by the council became vacant. These tended to be in the large estates built at Sandside and Leaside, Firth. This became a convenient dumping ground for homeless people; not the unfortunates who by fire, flood or otherwise had lost their homes, but the people who appeared from south with no place to go, forcing the local council to house them. How or why so many appeared in Shetland is unknown. At one time articles in the national press on the 'gold rush' attracted hundreds, but that period of plenty had now gone.

Family 'X' were the extreme of this migration, arriving as man, partner, and two children. They had no money and no possessions, relying entirely on the local authority to provide all and knowing every facet of the social security requirements. In fact, rumour had it that the man had a copy of their confidential regulations not normally allowed out of the office. This man boasted to us that he had rung the social security office in the town in Scotland they had come from thirty-nine times in one day and he soon became the constant headache of the local welfare office.

They were housed at Firth and the essentials provided including various electrical appliances such as a refrigerator. I mention these items because after six or seven months they suddenly departed but, before they left, they sold the house contents and equipped the entire family with leather jackets on the proceeds. No action seemed to be taken, and when a few weeks later they reappeared back in Shetland the same refurbishment of the house was undertaken.

Both man and woman were aggressive, abusive, manipulative, and forever quoting their rights with outright threats as to the action they would take if their demands were not met. They had, of course, no transport and refused to use the local bus service so demands for a doctor to visit were almost always in the evening. To make matters worse, the woman became pregnant and refused to attend the antenatal clinic at Brae in spite of all the efforts to persuade her it was for her own benefit.

The man put in calls for gastric bleeding frequently. Nothing was ever found on examination and no evidence of blood ever produced. This meant an emergency admission to hospital where he received something like pethidine or morphine, only to discharge himself the following morning. His medical notes when they arrived showed this was a common game in his last practice. We just had to go along with this charade as indeed the local hospital was forced to admit him knowing full well no proper investigation could be undertaken before he walked out.

The woman announced she was going to have a home confinement. When I said no, the conditions were not suitable, she lunged forward at me and I thought I was going to be physically as well as verbally assaulted.

One evening I was called because the man had fallen and hurt his back. I examined him very carefully and could find no evidence of any injury. I told him he had probably just bruised his back and I would leave him some analgesics. He demanded admission to hospital and I refused. He then demanded a second medical opinion. This, I advised him, was entirely his affair. That evening I had two further telephone calls from GPs in Shetland asking about the patient who had contacted them wanting a second opinion. When I explained the situation they wisely refused to attend. He obviously could get up to the phone when I left though he was flat on his back on the settee in simulated pain when I was there. He recovered very quickly but told the social worker he would 'have me' if it was the last thing he did. This warning from the social worker was nothing surprising to us as the veiled references to lawyers or the health board were common place. We knew how real the danger was but just had to live with it. To have them removed from our list and allocated to another doctor was useless as being the only doctors in the area they would have been reallocated to us. They probably were just as aware of the regulations as we were.

While the pregnancy progressed they decided to have a trip south. Where the money for fares came from is unknown. She went into labour prematurely south of Fair Isle necessitating a helicopter evacuation. Needless to say the labour had disappeared by the time she was admitted in Aberdeen. To make matters worse the media homed in and he enjoyed every minute of it.

One of the children was unwell and diabetes was found. This necessitated admission to Aberdeen with the state paying for father to attend. He then tried to make a case against us for failing to make the diagnosis earlier. Nothing came of that because there was no case to answer and I presume his lawyer had the sense to advise him. The child was so dirty and neglected on admission steps were set in motion by the authorities for both the children to be taken into care. We were not involved in that other than the attendance of myself at a care conference in Aberdeen, yet further expense for the state. The consultant stated quite definitely the child could not be treated properly at home for the diabetes. We were relieved and shortly after this the parents suddenly departed.

The last episode to this trying tale took place a year or so after they left. Somebody brought a newspaper cutting into the surgery of the man's wedding to another woman, not the one we knew.

There was a handful of other problem patients who could make life hell for a doctor by their incessant, untimely and unnecessary demands, but none came anywhere near the 'Xs'. I suppose 'X' did 'get' me as he had threatened in the end, for after two years of them I decided I would retire as soon as I could.

I could never have survived an inner city practice where tales of the type I have just illustrated are apparently everyday occurrences. When I thought about it, I think that if I had had to practice under these conditions I would have found any kind of job rather than thole it. Undoubtedly, I had been spoiled by my earlier years in practice.

A friend of mine in general practice in Johnston told me that a colleague of his had been called out to one of his patients at 11pm. When he got there the patient said, "It's not for one of us but for my father. He has missed the last bus home so we thought as you are always available you might run him home." The strange thing is that the doctor did just that, but removed the family from his list next day.

A medical partnership is like a marriage. Working together in such close proximity demands excellent co-operation, absolute reliability, and trust. It was only when employing locums if the other partner was away on holiday that I realised how much I depended on these qualities. It was sometimes tempting in the middle of the night to leave all the tidying up until the next day but it was not helpful for the partner to come in next morning to a mess. It is sometimes not easy to always agree on policy or the organisation of a practice but in fourteen years with Dawson we never had any disagreement of any kind however small. I could not have had a better colleague. The only subject where we agreed to differ was politics and as a result it was never discussed.

After I had retired, Dawson had little success in attracting a partner for some time but eventually got one. Dawson never complained to me though I knew and sensed that it was no longer the happy ship. Fate had a hand, however, in releasing him early from the practice, not the way one would have chosen, when he had a mild cardiac infarction. This resulted in an early medical retirement and he enjoyed five years retirement until cancer ended it. As he said himself, if he had not had the infarction he would have died in harness.

Over many years there had been a gradual erosion of general practice, mainly by government interference in the National Health Service. The amount of paperwork had trebled and became more important to the mushrooming administrators than the patients. This produced a power struggle and empire-building on a grand scale, with doctors having less and less say in both general practice and in hospital. It became very irritating when everything ended up in committees where often our advice was ignored, especially things we had practical experience of over many years.

Oh for the days of the Executive Council, John Johnston, John Shearer and Ina Hunter, with Davy Fotheringham as clerk of works. It was relatively easy to practice with so few administrators and who knew the job inside out.

Some years ago all the dispensing doctors in Shetland used non-proprietary drugs in their practices, saving the NHS many thousands of pounds. The government decided to assess GPs' drug costs then to allocate an amount for drugs based on that assessment. To overspend meant an enquiry and if no good explanation could be found a fine of some sort could be imposed. The result of this was we all changed to proprietary preparations in the months preceding the assessment to inflate the drug budget, thereby giving ourselves a margin. Needless to say many proprietaries were continued instead of going back to the less expensive preparations simply because it was easier for patients on long term prescriptions to continue with exactly the same size, type, and colour of tablet. To revert back caused yet another explanation as to why the specific tablet was slightly different and reassurance that it did exactly the same job as the previous one. Some were never convinced that a new tablet was as good as the old one.

Chapter 28

Dogs

DOGS have played their part in my life in various ways. I have related various attempts to practice veterinary medicine in the Unst years and how I was the victim of their teeth twice.

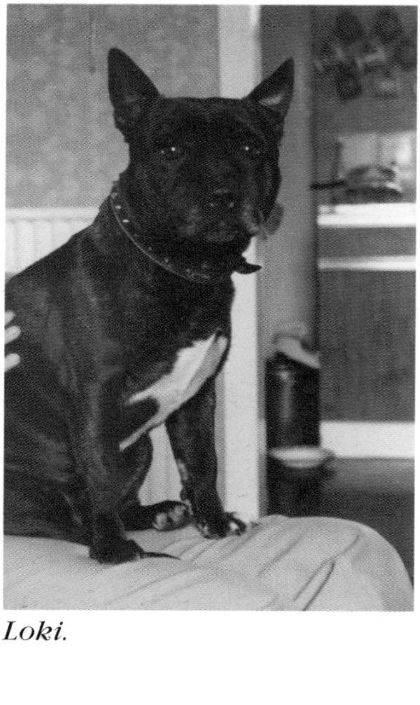

Loki.

Having enjoyed Dr Porter's Bill, the Staffordshire bull terrier, so much, we acquired our own after we were settled in Unst. We had two dogs, Rasmie then Loki, then our daughter Jane gave us the present of a bitch, Hekla, when she got married and wanted a Staffie for herself; hers was called Rasmie too and I have never seen such a good natured dog.

At one period we looked after Rasmie and I took him up to the surgery with me in the morning. He was tied to the radiator behind my desk and just lay there during surgery enjoying the heat as all bull terriers do.

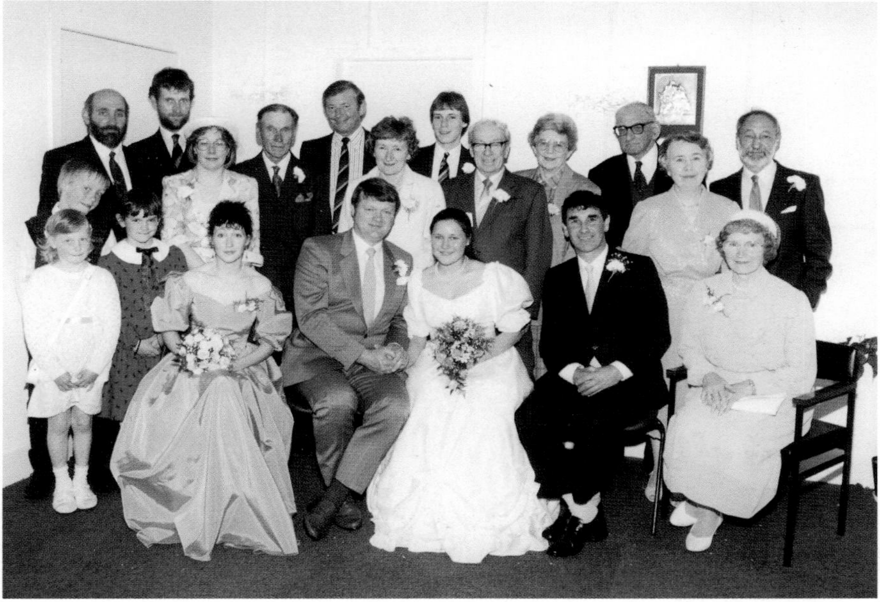

Jane and Peter's wedding, 1988. Back (from left): Eric Fillmore, David Manson, Susan Manson, Peter Manson (senior), John Gamble (Maureen's brother), Olive Livings (Maureen's sister), John Robertson, Harry Livings, Betty Haddon (Maureen's sister), Lindsay Robertson, Margaret Robertson, the author. Front: Gregor Manson, Jane Manson, Jessie Fillmore, Susan Robertson, Peter Manson, Jane, Bill Kirkpatrick, Maureen Robertson.

The dog could not be seen from the patient's side of the desk so it was very amusing for me when he snorted or grunted as he was prone to do when sleeping. If you know your patients well, and can judge when to lighten the normally serious business of a consultation, these peculiar noises could be very funny.

One lady whom I knew was full of fun proceeded to explain her medical problem. I listened carefully. Suddenly Rasmie snorted and she stopped in mid-sentence, looking at me intently, but as I said nothing and kept a straight face she proceeded with her story. On the third snort she stopped again and asked, "What was that?"

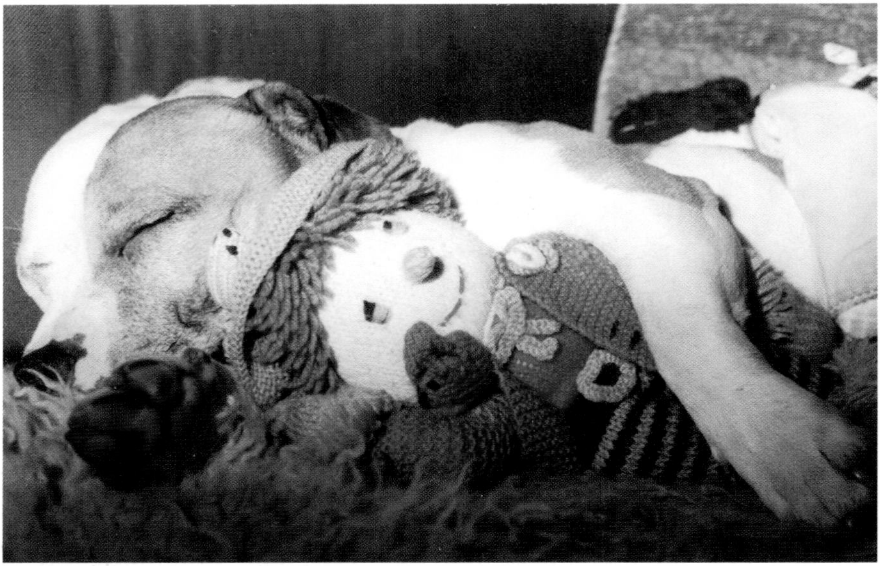

Jane's Rasmie with companion.

"What was what?" I replied.

"A funny snoring type of noise," she said.

"Oh, that," I suddenly seemed to catch on, "I always make that noise when I am considering a diagnosis."

She looked at me strangely for a moment then seemed to accept it, proceeding in spite of further strange noises to complete her story. Only when she was about to leave the consulting room did I take her over to look behind the desk. She enjoyed the joke as much as I did and as indeed I knew she would.

When I did not know the patient well enough I had to explain it was the dog and display him. Poor fellow, I had to tie him up to stop him greeting everybody who came into the room. Some people don't like dogs and are especially anxious about bull terriers who look a bit fierce.

On the other hand, Rasmie sometimes proved a great asset when the patient was a child. It helped to distract them from any necessary examination.

Chapter 29

Retiral

'R'DAY – April the sixth, 1992 – was gradually getting nearer but there was still some serious business to come. The first of these was a standard request for a visit to a young girl in one of the farther reaches of the practice. She had been unwell during the night with a temperature. When I examined her I knew that I was seeing my first case of meningitis ever. Fortunately Dr Clubb and I had carried for years a specific intra muscular antibiotic for meningitis. It had gone out of date and been renewed frequently in our black bags over the years, seemingly an expensive whim on our part. All that meant nothing now that it was required. The patient was immediately transferred to Aberdeen by air ambulance and I am glad to say never looked back.

Peter Peterson's advice about appendicitis or meningitis had at last borne fruit.

Approaching the end of thirty-three years in general practice all doctors I am sure wish for a quiet non-eventful exit. However, the sudden call into the unknown, usually during the night when you were very much alone, was an ever-present anxiety. And so it was almost at the end of my contract. Wakened suddenly by the phone always produced some palpitations, a dry mouth and frantic attempts to clear the soporific fog, and engage the neutral cerebral cells in gear. This latter problem often necessitated a request to repeat name, address, etc., thereby giving a few extra seconds to switch on.

"This is Mrs 'so-&-so', there's been a fight and I think he's dead!" This message at 1am dispelled the sleepy mists in a flash. Murder was the last thing I expected or wanted but that was what I was now involved in.

On arrival at the house there was a very subdued husband and wife and a battered man. Examination quickly proved that he was dead. Not only was it a rare event for Shetland but to make matters worse, both men were ex-patients of mine from Unst. The next stage was to bring in the police before further examining the body. It was almost breakfast time by the time I got away from the scene. There followed reports to be furnished and worst of all a summons to the High Court in Aberdeen.

This is an unpleasant experience for anybody and I had had one previous appearance at the Court of Session in Edinburgh when I was in Unst. In that case it was a divorce case, but both

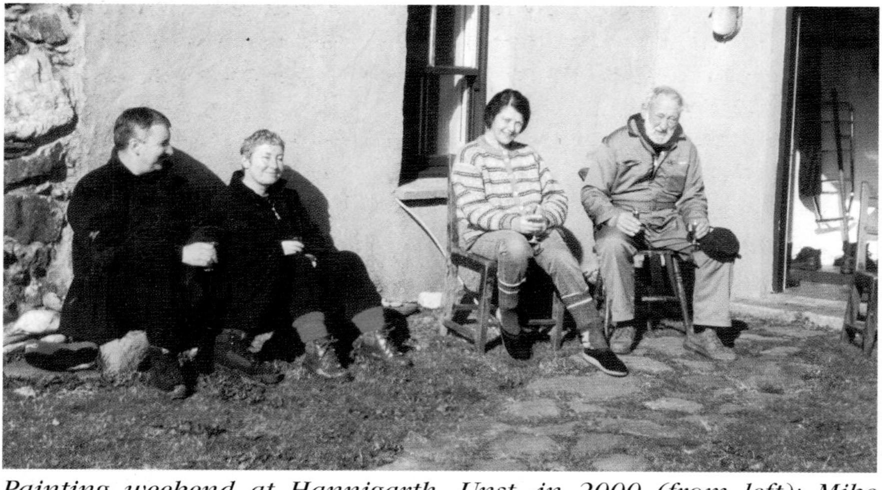

Painting weekend at Hannigarth, Unst, in 2000 (from left): Mike Finnie, Anne Bain, June Redman, the author.

being patients when I came to confidential medical questions I had to ask the judge how I was placed. He instructed me to divulge the appropriate facts. Having answered Counsel I was allowed to leave the court, the whole thing apart from waiting most of the morning, only took about ten minutes.

Fortunately at the court in Aberdeen, having waited all morning to be called, the witnesses were suddenly allowed as a group into court. The accused had changed his plea to guilty at the last moment so we would not be required as witnesses but were given the doubtful privilege to attend sentence. The charge had been reduced and the sentence followed suit. I found a travel agent in Union Street just opposite the court house immediately the case was over and by 4pm was on my way back to Shetland.

It all ended on a high note. Firstly a presentation from the community council of a superb music centre and a picture mount cutter, both in constant use today, and then an invitation to Busta House for a party and what a first class party it turned out to be. Initially, however, I thought this is a very badly organised event as we were very forcibly told to attend at seven o'clock on the dot. I wondered about this briefly but dismissed it. On arrival there were only four or five people there and nobody to organise drinks. We were next told to sit in a particular seat and to remain in it. By this time I was becoming a bit mesmerised but did as I was bid.

What I did not know was that various people had been secretly arriving after seven o'clock and that our enforced seating arrangements meant we had our backs to the steps and the entrance.

Dawson and the practice nurses had arranged a 'This is Your Life' book and like rabbits out of a hat, produced Liz Munro from Aberdeen, our first practice nurse, Kay Naisbitt from York, our second recruit, and thereafter many friends. It was the most pleasant surprise I have ever had.

There was lots of other foolery as the evening went on with much hilarity, splendid company and good food. The whole evening was a pleasurable haze of conviviality.

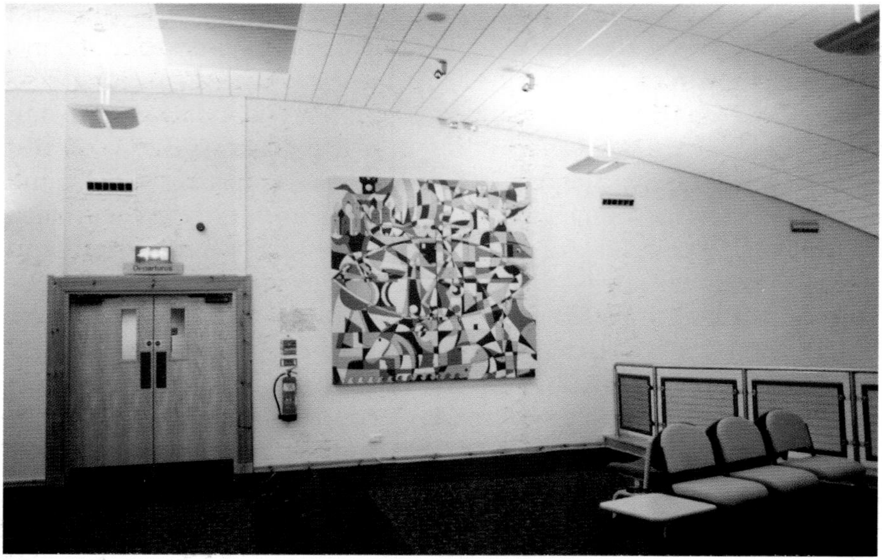

The painting designed for Lerwick Port Authority, in the ferry terminal.

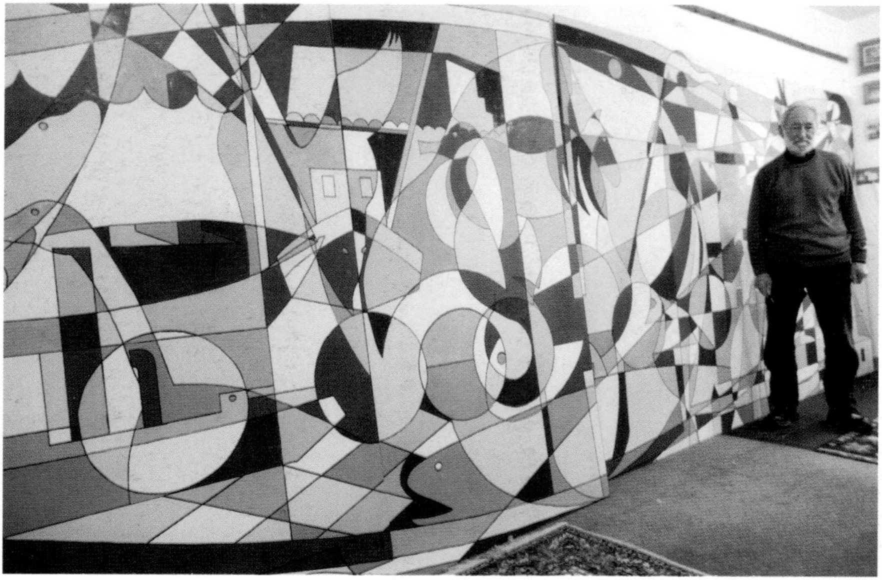

Two-thirds of completed mural for the Norröna.

I thought that was it and I could hang up my stethoscope and get on the boilersuit. However, I went back for a couple of days after Dawson had his heart attack to help out and a year or so later agreed to fill a short vacancy in Unst when Dr Karam was in hospital. Since then I have let my medical protection and registration with the General Medical Council lapse so became unable to practice. For some years I used to pop into the health centre to make sure the girls were behaving but as fewer and fewer of the old guard remained this has gradually lapsed.

And what about retirement? The only thing that worries me a little is that I might waken up some morning and say to myself, "What am I going to do today?" So far it has never happened. I saw many men who had to retire at retiral age who had no real interest outside their occupation who lived only a year or two and then died. I often wondered if it was like some people in Africa that I have heard of who just turned their faces to the wall and decided to die. Psychological factors are no doubt important

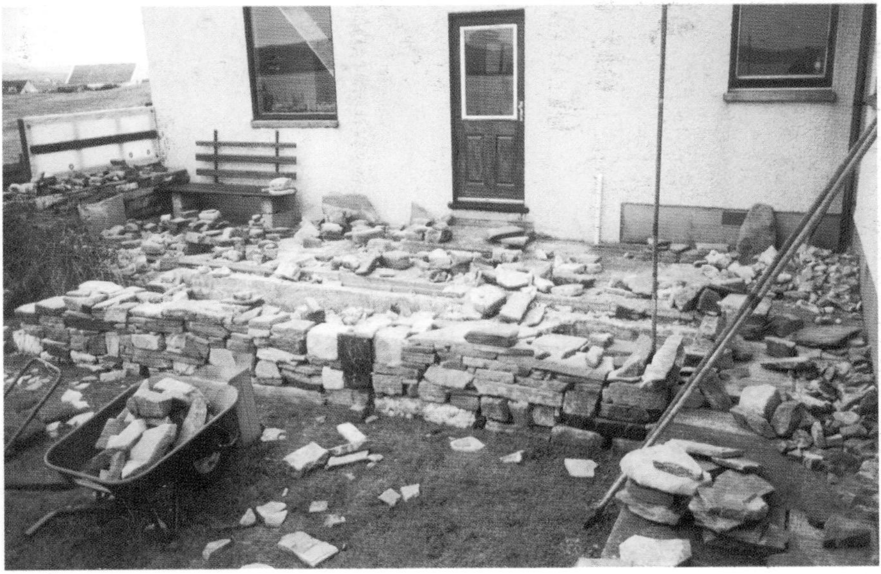

Drystone dyke in progress at Fjaere.

in these cases brought on by boredom, a feeling of uselessness and thus a lack of motivation to live.

My advice to anyone approaching retirement is make sure you have as many projects lined up as possible and make sure they are both inside and outside pursuits to accommodate the worst of the Shetland weather.

If all else fails I quite enjoy getting the vacuum cleaner out. This is in keeping with my mildly obsessive compulsive personality.

Speaking to colleagues in practice over the last few years has convinced me that I did the right thing to retire when I did. More and more GPs I speak to bemoan the decline of the NHS which has been suffocated by bureaucracy and throttled with paperwork. I fear we are watching the death throes of the NHS, a service I spent my working life in and firmly believed in in its original form. American litigation spreading to the UK and human frailty have completed the prescription.